DATE DUE

3118296	'JUL 0 7 1998

Community Health Psychology

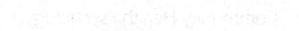

Community Health Psychology
Empowerment for Diverse Communities

Victor De La Cancela,
Jean Lau Chin, and Yvonne M. Jenkins

Foreword by J. Emilio Carrillo

Routledge
New York   London

Published in 1998 by
Routledge
29 West 35th Street
New York, NY 10001

Published in Great Britain by
Routledge
11 New Fetter Lane
London EC4P 4EE

Library of Congress Cataloging-in-Publication Data
De La Cancela, Victor.
    Community health psychology : empowerment for diverse communities
  /   Victor De La Cancela, Jean Lau Chin, Yvonne M. Jenkins : foreword by
  Emilio Carrilo.
        p.   cm.
    Includes bibliographical references and index.
    ISBN 0-415-91426-4 (hbk.). — ISBN 0-415-91427-2 (pbk.)
        1. Minorities—Medical care—United States. 2. Community health
  services—United States. 3. Transcultural medical care—United
  States. I. Chin, Jean Lau. II. Jenkins, Yvonne M., 1952–   .
  III. Title.
  RA448.4.C66 1997
  362.1´089´00978—DC21   97-21660
                                                                          CIP

DEDICATION

I, Victor De La Cancela, dedicate this book to my family and friends for their patience and love, to Corrinne for her love, support, encouragement and sacrifice, and my in-laws for enriching my life with theirs; and to "mi querida hija" Elena Cameron for being. I especially dedicate this book to the memory of my dad, Luis Fernandez De La Cancela, a Puerto Rican "independentista" and a merchant marine who died tragically on the last voyage before his retirement. His internal injuries from a shipboard accident in waters outside of Chile were not attended to due to barriers to care posed by the United States' political differences with Salvador Allende's socialist government. May a people's sociopolitical, economic, and cultural struggle against oppression never be used to deny the sick humane health care.

I, Jean Lau Chin, dedicate this book to the underserved communities among ethnic minority populations and especially Asian American immigrants and refugees who have been unable to access care because of language and cultural barriers. I also dedicate this book to my family for their support, to South Cove Community Health Center for their continued advocacy to improve access to health care for Asian Americans, and lastly to my mother Fung Gor Lee, an immigrant, who symbolized the barriers faced by Asian Americans in utilizing the health care system.

I, Yvonne M. Jenkins, dedicate this book to the memory of my grandparents: Alona, Lanie, and Alonzo who died before I was born, and whose lives ended painfully, tragically, and prematurely after being denied health care as a consequence of prejudice and racial discrimination. I also dedicate this book to grandpa Thomas whom I had the privilege of knowing for a short while before he, too, quietly slipped away out of despair. May social ills never again prevail over the basic human right to secure quality health care. Finally, with much joy I dedicate this book to Ylana Janet, my most beloved and precious gift, with much love and hope for a healthy and happy future.

Contents

Foreword

J. Emilio Carrillo

In the midst of the managed care revolution and the tumultuous rush of conversions of nonprofit hospitals and health plans to for-profit status, a voice calls out for a more empowering and consumer centered health care system. The authors of *Community Health Psychology: Empowerment for Diverse Communities* call for a health care system that seeks to improve health, not generate wealth. They call for an analysis of health problems and systems that is based on an integration of social, psychological, and cultural factors, rather than a more limited, dichotomized, predominantly biomedical perspective. Solutions are at the community level and are rooted in prevention and public health.

Clearly, these are not the concerns that are driving the current blind rush to a new version of the U.S. health care "patchwork quilt." Unlike much of the rest of the world, the health care processes in our country have traditionally lacked the forethought, coherence, and comprehensiveness necessary to be considered a true health care system. Instead, an irrationally constructed amalgam of employment-based insurance, entitlement programs for a fraction of the poor with great interstate variations, and an insufficient program for the elderly (as well as a callous disregard of the needs of the "uninsured" and total neglect of "illegal aliens") characterize the past of U.S. health care, a past which is currently under siege by powerful new market forces.

The escalating health care costs in the 1960s and 1970s provided fertile ground for entrepreneurs to devise ways by which the rate of rising health care costs could be checked by shifting costs while still carving out a handsome profit. The ascendancy of the new intermediary, the managed care company, resulted in huge hospital mergers and the formation of physician networks which could not have been imagined just a few years earlier. Hospitals and physicians thus attempted to again deal directly with the payors, large employers and the government programs of Medicaid and Medicare, and eliminate the go-between man who was now making the big profits. Meanwhile, what about the poor and disenfranchised? Managed care companies have grown even richer by not having to contribute to the education of physicians nor so called "charity care." The economic survival of municipal and public hospitals has become seriously threatened by cost and profit shifting, while the rapidly growing chains of for-profit hospitals have cornered the market in many parts of the country. The higher administrative costs and profit margins in these for-profit hospitals leave little room for the care of the uninsured.

As health care becomes a financial game with higher financial stakes, the question of who cares for the poor and the uninsured becomes even more daunting. While the putative answer would seem to be the government, the health care reform efforts of President and Mrs. Clinton were stymied by the well-placed dollars of the powerful health insurance lobby. The Health Security Act could not survive even in a democratically controlled Congress.

We should not forget that this legislation, which sought to provide health insurance for "all Americans" by creating a regulated yet competitive environment for the health care industry, did not provide coverage for millions of immigrants. Current bipartisan efforts at the federal and state levels to incrementally provide expanded health insurance coverage and regulate the managed care industry are diffuse and incoherent. As the Medicaid rolls swell from the increased numbers of the "unemployed-uninsured," very realistic threats arise that the Medicaid program will be capped off. While the president of a leading managed care company amassed approximately half a billion dollars in 1995, families who don't qualify must do without needed medications. It doesn't seem that the government is ready to provide the kind of advocacy and financial support that the poor and disenfranchised require.

The authors of *Community Health Psychology* envision a higher quality of care. They propose "a community health psychology perspective to look at health needs, health status, and systems of health

care to effect change, and to promote access and cultural competence within systems of care so that they can more effectively serve
the diversity within all communities." (Aims and Scope, p. 000).
During the debate of the Clinton plan just a few years ago, the discussion centered on universal coverage and cost containment, and
little was said about quality of care. The debate on quality has been
framed by the managed care industry—not government, not even the
medical and public health professional societies. The National Committee for Quality Assurance (NCQA) was formed in 1979 through a
joint effort of the principal managed care trade associations. The
NCQA develops performance measures for plans through the Health
Plan Employer Data and Information Set (HEDIS). These quality
standards have been embraced by the entire managed care industry
and even by government. The State of New York has recently
adopted the HEDIS (Version 3.0) as its principal quality indicator for
its Medicaid Managed Care program. The quality of care of a largely
Latino/a and African American Medicaid-insured population in
New York will be derived from standards developed by a corporate
culture with little, if any, relationship to the diverse cultures described in this book. Needless to say, HEDIS has no standards for a
human behavior that is "holistic and inclusive of physical and psychological health" (Aims and Scope, p. 1) nor does it explore the
clinical and institutional barriers to service delivery which are listed
in Table 9.1 (Chapter 9, p. 228). Sadly, just as the victors of war write
the history books, so do those who control the health care capital
write the rules of quality assurance.

The authors of *Community Health Psychology: Empowerment for
Diverse Communities* provide a vision of a more complete, more
human system of care. They understand that health is not simply
determined by the function of a particular gene or enzyme, but by a
complex interaction of environment and self, body and mind, society and community. They understand that what they describe does
not come easy, but that the vision of the whole can help inform the
small steps that health care providers must take every day.

AIMS AND SCOPE

What Is Community Health Psychology?: Empowerment for Diverse Communities

Victor De La Cancela, Jean Lau Chin, Yvonne M. Jenkins

With the rapid growth of people of color within the U.S. population, few models have enabled us to effectively address the different needs and health services required by diverse communities. Many existing models look at health as an individual issue, that is, what services an individual needs, and how healthy he or she is. Many use a "bell curve" or "normal" assumption in looking at needs, status, and service delivery in attempting to influence the health of the majority of the population, that is, how do we reach the most people? The influence of current models of health policy, public health, and health care administration has often served to exclude and disempower communities of color. As a result, communities of color have remained underserved; their health needs have not been met within "mainstream" service delivery systems. These models have led to disparities in health status among communities of color as compared to those for Caucasian communities, i.e., a comparative model which only examines those needs and those statuses which are disparate from a white standard. These models have also posted obstacles to gaining access to services since many systems of care incompetently address the cultural, linguistic, and financial barriers communities of color experience in utilizing and gaining entry to health care services.

We intend to describe a community health psychology model which will enable psychologists, administrators, and health service providers to contribute to health policy, public health, and health care administration which is relevant to our evolving and increasingly diverse society.

As psychologists enhancing the understanding of human behavior, we see the need to include multiple bio-psycho-politico and social contexts in our formulations. We understand individuals to behave within family, community, societal, and political contexts, as well as with intrapsychic contexts, which shape human health. We cannot speak of individual health status without recognizing the pernicious, external stressors that routinely deplete rather than enhance community resources. Familiar examples are poverty, violence, racism, and substance abuse. We view human behavior as holistic and inclusive of physical, social, and psychological health. Psychological health involves acknowledgment of the influences of chronic illness (i.e., cancer, hypertension), infectious disease (i.e., HIV/AIDS), transmission of illness (i.e., sickle cell anemia, thalassemia), *and* societal and institutional pathologies (i.e., racism, prejudice), internalized oppression (i.e., intragroup violence), and environmental factors (i.e., substandard housing, inadequate public schools, routine exposure to toxic waste) on individual health and the well-being of our communities. It is our contention that systems of health care must respond not only to the needs and health status of individuals, but also must be shaped by a wider perspective of the communities in which these individuals live.

Hence, we expand the definition of psychology to be inclusive of health and community. We look at health in terms of a triadic interaction of health needs, health status, and systems of health care impacting a specific community. Community can be defined as individuals who share certain commonalities, be they cultural or geographic, social or political. In this context, the larger society refers to the Caucasian middle class which has been the dominant group in the United States.

We propose a community health psychology perspective to look at health needs, health status, and systems of health care to effect change, and to promote access and cultural competence within systems of care so that they can more effectively serve the diversity within all communities. We are particularly interested in this perspective being inclusive of communities of color who have been historically underserved and marginalized by models which define health primarily in biomedical terms. Our question is: How do we serve all people? We are particularly interested in community health psychology as a change agent and focus this change on systemic levels via policy, administration, and health education and advocacy.

Consequently, we approach questions about health and community from the sociopolitical, community, and cultural contexts which impact our systems of health care delivery. Because we emphasize a community perspective, our questions include: How does the community define health? How healthy is the community in which the individual lives? What systems of care are needed to reach all segments of the population? Our approach is integrative of communities of color but differential in respecting and maintaining as significant their differences in needs, perspectives, and origins.

The community health psychology perspective is intended to promote change via policy development, administration, and public health. The intended outcomes are the improved health of a community, empowerment for communities of color, and improved access and cultural competence in our systems of care. A key concept of the community health psychology perspective is a diversity orientation which is inclusive, systemic, culturally competent, and comprehensive in its approach. By diversity, we mean the acknowledgement and valuing of differences, the acceptance and utilization of these in identifying needs, measuring health status, and designing systems of health care delivery. By inclusive, we mean the inclusion of all segments of the population, especially communities of color who have been historically underserved. By systemic, we mean a recognition of community, administrative, regulatory, policy, and other factors which influence and interact with individual health behavior and service utilization, and an emphasis on a community-based approach to service delivery. By cultural competence, we mean the ability of providers and systems of health care at all levels to meet the needs of all segments of the population, that is, a service delivery system that is effective in addressing the needs of the specific community in the context of its cultural beliefs, values, language, practices, and health behaviors. By comprehensive, we mean a total health emphasis that goes beyond the individual doctor-patient relationship, and is inclusive of health education and promotion; prevention; community outreach; and adequate transitional programs for deinstitutionalized patients, prisoners, survivors, and consumers from acute care facilities, jails, psychiatric hospitals, and custodial developmental disabilities centers. In sum, a community health psychology perspective can help to promote change via policy, administration, community education, and advocacy to ensure competence and promote access for all segments of the population.

Using this community health psychology perspective, the key concepts identified above guide the organization of chapters in the book. Section I examines our communities. Chapters 1 and 2 focus on population diversity and needs of communities of color, while Chapter 3 discusses differential manifestation of health status within communities of color. Section II examines our systems of health care and recommends approaches to improve them. Chapter 4 describes systemic issues of health care delivery from a macro and administrative level, while Chapter 5 discusses systemic issues from a micro and provider level.

We then move to individual approaches to change by each of the authors in the following three chapters, capturing our multiple and interacting perspectives within three different systems of care: municipal health system, community health center, and university health services. These include our views of individual and community health; our roles as administrator and provider, our roles as policymakers and as "survivors" or consumers of the system. We also include our roles as psychologists in health care systems; our views of health, which link mind and body; the perception of our settings as private and public systems of care, community and "mainstream"; and our ability to empower through effecting change from inside or outside the "mainstream" system. These dyadic views capture the diversity of systems and roles which contribute to our formulations of a community health psychology perspective. They provide a historical and developmental perspective, through individual case studies, to currents in health care reform and community mental health.

We end with Section III, Toward New Models, to highlight our conclusions for health policy and public health. We view prevention as a focus to improve the health of different communities using different approaches. Current movements in health care promise to change the scope of our systems of care. Disparities both in health status, and access to quality health service will remain unless policymakers and administrators arm themselves with models of diversity and cultural competence to shape the regulations and priorities which influence health and health care delivery. We hope to transform the roles of psychologists, administrators, and policymakers through a community health psychology perspective.

SECTION I

HEALTH STATUS AND NEEDS OF DIVERSE COMMUNITIES

Henry Tomes

Community Health Psychology: Empowerment for Diverse Communities is a book that is many years, probably decades, overdue. This opening section, "Health Status and Needs of Diverse Communities" looks at complex interactions between health and illness as they are conditioned by individual, group, community, and cultural factors. The chapters that make up Section I delineate issues of health care needs, health systems reform, and the psychosocial and cultural impact on health status. However, these chapters raise the important questions of why and how the health status of people of color has been neglected and ways in which that neglect can be overcome. First, why?

Demographers have predicted that by 2050 there will be no racial or ethnic majority group within the United States. Latinos/as, African Americans, Asian Americans, and American Indians[1] as a group will equal or surpass European Americans in sheer numbers. While European Americans will no longer be in the majority, they will still constitute the largest ethnic group. The Latino/a population will have passed African Americans as the second largest group. The Asian American population will continue its growth, surpassing that of American Indians.

The "why" indicated above is answered in the section chapters which catalog requirements of a health system capable of providing effective care to all of its citizens, not just those of European deriva-

---

1. With the exception of Dr. Pamela Jumper Thurman's commentary on Chapter Two, the health status and needs of American Indians are not addressed in this section.

tion. When one looks at the health status of people of color and determines what needs to be done and how long it will take, at least 50 years of concerted, good-faith effort will be required at a minimum to effect the social and educational changes needed to provide culturally competent and technologically effective health and behavioral health systems.

"Why" is also addressed by examining ways in which community and cultural factors impact the ways persons of color, specific to their own communities, see health, illness, disease, and treatment. This early section does not deny the effectiveness and efficiency of organized medicine, rather it goes to great length to illustrate how Western providers can become able to understand how individuals interpret their bodily dysfunctions within a community context. Special emphasis is placed on the sick role and how a diagnosis may not motivate a search for and compliance with effective treatment, but instead may lead to the assumption of a preordained outcome unrelated to reduction or removal of symptoms. Throughout these early chapters, explanations are offered which permit the reader to understand ways in which cultural missteps occur when persons with different cultural understandings communicate past each other when the intent is, on the one hand, to give what is needed, and, on the other, to receive what is needed.

While the "why" of health status is rooted in historical and cultural beliefs and behaviors and the concomitant responses to modern medicine as presently practiced, the "how" requires change and adaptation to change within the health care system. To effect needed change, providers need an understanding of health-related behaviors that encompasses social, psychological, cultural, and specific ethnic issues related to health. The authors propose a community health psychology in which emphasis is placed on mastery of Western health interventions and technologies with meanings being attributed to them from an array of contextual variables.

Contextual variables such as language are usually accepted as providing meaning, with meaning being conveyed by idioms, dialects, etc., within the frame of linguistic convention. No matter how skilled the practitioner, failure to develop effective communication skills leads to ineffective interventions with individuals and within communities. Emphasis is placed, correctly so, on subtleties within groups. For instance, within the Latino/a community, Spanish speakers must also be understood within their sociocultural contexts. Recent articles and discussions in the popular media focusing on Ebonics in African American communities and Spanglish in certain Latino/a communities demonstrate even further the dynamic and changing manner of speaking and understanding.

However complex linguistic issues may seem for competent community health psychologists, they appear almost inconsequential when one begins to explore understandings of cultural factors which impinge on health status. Understandings of bodily functions, the importance of food and eating, beliefs about sex and reproductive processes, and beliefs about illness and health challenge the effective provision of health care. When such health care is mental health care, the culturally competent provider is essential.

Mental and emotional disorders continue to provide challenges to public and private mental health systems. When sociocultural matters are factored in, the design and implementation of culturally appropriate mental health care becomes even more daunting. Appropriate and effective care provides opportunities for persons experiencing a range of symptoms from mild discomfort to disabling psychoses to receive care that facilitates functioning. While psychiatric medications provide symptomatic relief for some, for others even the ingesting of such powerful medications has a distinct cultural flavor. It may be difficult to accept medications when patients themselves and those around them believe psychological difficulties to arise from malevolent external forces. Such cultural underpinnings explain the large number of missed appointments and other noncompliant behaviors that bedevil therapists who treat those whose belief systems contain significant folk and spiritual influences. So not only do community health psychologists need a mixture of understandings to effect positive interventions, they will also encounter ongoing evaluation and research opportunities, some of which may be of an ethnographic nature.

1

Health Care Needs of Communities of Color

Victor De La Cancela,
Jean Lau Chin, and Yvonne M. Jenkins

To develop a community health psychology perspective, we need first to understand the health research findings and advocacy positions related to the health and human service needs and demographic trends of U.S. communities of color. We propose a comprehensive and systemic approach which emphasizes interorganizational planning, collaboration and coalition building among disenfranchised communities, multidisciplinary programming, grassroots organizing, and community health education. We will examine, in turn, the diverse health needs of Latino/a, Asian American, and African American persons and present different approaches to prevention and community-based health care.

While diversity and differences exist within and between communities of color, some crosscutting issues bond their perspectives. It is imperative to identify these themes to mobilize us toward models of community empowerment and cultural competence. A holistic approach to health needs, health care, and health reform is one theme, and is captured in the integration of mind, body, and spirit found important among communities of color. Community networks and the importance of cultural values and beliefs in health care practices and identification of health needs are another. Lastly, the disenfranchisement felt by communities of color is a theme reflecting the institutional and individual racism which pose barriers to full participation in the economic and social opportunities of U.S. society.

As community-based service organizations prepare to meet the challenges of the twenty-first century, changes in national and regional population demographics and utilization trends will have implications for program and service development strategies. As resources shrink, community-based organizations will compete with large, established "mainstream" service agencies for scarce resources. As the ethnic and racial make-up of the country changes, with people of color making up 35% of the U.S. population by the year 2000 according to Census projections, both large and small health and human-service agencies will need to set directions to better position their organizations and to achieve a mission which is inclusive of communities of color. As managed care grows, there will be a growing concern regarding how to provide high-quality, cost-effective health services to communities of color.

Communities of color in the United States have diverse migration and immigration patterns, cultural and religious values, adaptation experiences and health care needs coupled with unique intergroup relations related to race, population settlement patterns in the United States, and sociopolitical histories. This diversity includes undocumented and legal immigrants, migrant and disenfranchised U.S. citizens in the continental United States, in Puerto Rico, and in U.S. territories within the Pacific. Unfortunately, this diversity within and among communities of color has been masked when planners lump all Latinos/as, Asian Americans, or African Americans into a national, singular category that hides the specific social problems of subgroups and makes it politically difficult to demonstrate need and positively change the quality of life for underserved communities.

CUERPO, MENTE, Y ESPIRITU: HEALTHY PRAXIS WITH LATINOS/AS

We have selectively reviewed both the generic and specific Latino/a subgroup health and human services needs literature and health policy research literature. This review provides a framework for more progressive, comprehensive, and timely community-based health psychology praxis with Latinos/as. While much of it has applications for other communities of color, our focus on Latinos/as serves to preserve the uniqueness of need and approaches that are important for a culturally competent service delivery system. We proceed from a body, mind, and spirit (*cuerpo, mente, y espiritu*) integrative perspective or holistic approach to health services delivery.

In this context *espiritu* refers to a sought-after cooperative spirit that involves networking, collaboration, inclusion, linkages, technical assistance, service recipient, and community representation and input, community self-help and empowerment, and local community development.

Our review and discussion focuses on community health psychology because Latinos/as do not typically engage in mind-body dualism in referring to personal, family, and community health. More often than not, *salud* (health) in the Latino/a context refers to health status, quality of life issues, and a self-healing, spiritual or religious orientation with positive health practices (De La Cancela, 1989). Our intent is to encourage readers to ally with this familial, cultural, and truly biopsychosocial world view toward joining with Latino/a communities in their healing efforts.

Health Status and Needs

A multiservice, community-informed practice is critical to meeting the divergent health and human services needs of Latino/a subpopulations, that is, Puerto Rican, Cuban, Mexican, and Central and South American in the United States. Problems include the structural characteristics of the U.S. health care delivery system that discourage use by people in the lower socioeconomic classes, such as a lack of primary care physicians in large inner cities, inadequate transportation, and other travel difficulties. Another access problem is the rotating staff and dehumanizing features of public hospitals and clinics which have been found to impact particularly on Puerto Ricans (Schur et al., 1987). Using the 1977 National Medical Care Expenditure Survey, researchers found that 39% of Puerto Ricans go to a hospital outpatient clinic or emergency department to receive medical care, as compared to 31% of African Americans, 20% of Cuban Americans, and 9% of Caucasians.

A recent Northeast Hispanic Needs Conference convened by the ASPIRA Institute for Policy Research found the major health and human service needs of Latinos/as in Connecticut, Massachusetts, New Jersey, New York, and Rhode Island to be in the areas of: substance abuse, health education, financial access to health services, AIDS, teenage pregnancy, and domestic violence (Petrovich, 1987). Conference participants suggested that substance abuse prevention should focus on the earliest ages possible. They called for comprehensive health education approaches targeting all family age groups. Culture- and language-appropriate, developmental and multidisciplinary family centered information, education, prevention, and case management activities were suggested. Also recommended were increasing the availability of public transportation, babysitting and child care services, and the number of school and community health clinics.

In the area of community economic development and political participation, conference attendees identified major limitations to achievement of Latino/a empowerment in the Northeast due to insufficient leadership development vehicles. They identified needs for: developing the fundraising abilities of current and future Latino/a leaders; simplification of registration and voting procedures; developing Latino/a voters' capabilities in expressing concerns to policymakers and public officials; establishing coalitions with similarly concerned groups to effect change; increasing Latino/a representation in corporate and foundation policymaking boards; creating corporate mentoring programs to train Latinos/as for mid-level management roles; promoting for-profit arms of community-based organizations as a means to increase the fiscal autonomy of existing agencies; training for Latino/a community agency staff in communication and marketing; promoting the development of leadership skills for Latino/a youth; bringing Latino/a agencies together to engage in priorities determination, strategic planning, collaboration, and mutual support.

The Hispanic HANES (Health and Nutrition Examination Survey), conducted by the National Center for Health Statistics, indicates that 45% of Puerto Ricans, 40% of Mexicans and 63% of Cubans living in the continental United States, with diabetes, are unaware that they have the disease (Flega et al., 1985). Latina women are three times more likely than non-Latina Caucasian women to receive prenatal care late or not at all (Ventura, 1987). Other studies report that the health profiles of midwestern seasonal and migrant Latino/a farmworkers represent agrarian "third world" conditions including malnutrition and infectious and parasitic diseases (Dever, 1989). Compared to the general population, migrants generate more clinic visits for diabetes, medical supervision of infants and children, middle ear infection, pregnancy, hypertension, contact dermatitis, and eczema. Dental disease is the number one health problem for migrant children aged 10 to 14, and it also is the number one health problem for migrant males. Pregnancy is the most frequent presenting condition for migrant females ages 15 to 19. Males from 20 to 29 years visit clinics primarily for contact dermatitis and eczema, strep throat, scarlet fever, and dental problems. For male and female migrant and seasonal farmworkers in the 30 to 44, 45 to 64, and elderly age groups, two of the most common problems are diabetes and hypertension.

The American Medical Association's (AMA) Council on Scientific Affairs concluded that Latinos/as are at greater risk than the general public for tuberculosis, HIV infection, alcoholism, cirrhosis, specific cancers, and violent deaths (Coalition of Hispanic Health and Human Organizations, 1991). Death due to stomach cancer is twice as high for Latinos/as as for non-Latino/a Caucasians, and the incidence of female cervical cancers is also twice as high, although Latinas' survival rates slightly exceed those of non-Latina Caucasians. Mexican males have a 40% higher death risk from cirrhosis of the liver than non-Latino Caucasians. Homicide mortality rates among Puerto Rican, Cuban, and Mexican American male youth exceed non-Latino Caucasian male rates. Puerto Rican males have higher homicide death rates than African Americans and, along with Cuban males, they surpass Caucasian males' suicide rate. The 1987 homicide rate per 100,000 population for Latino males 15 to 34 years old was 53.1 compared to a homicide rate of 8.5 for the total U. S. population (Council on Scientific Affairs, 1991). Among Latino/a children and adolescents, gang-related homicide and legal intervention is the fourth leading cause of death in the one to fourteen years age range (Herrell, 1994). The reported incidence rate of tuberculosis is five times higher for Latinos/as than it is for non-Latino/a Caucasians (Jereb, et al., 1991).

The AMA Council on Scientific Affairs found that Puerto Ricans to reported the most chronic and acute medical conditions. The Hispanic HANES survey, which includes taking blood pressure, indicates that almost half of the Puerto Ricans surveyed with hypertension were not aware they had it. Puerto Ricans also have the highest infant mortality attributed to low birth weight. The renowned health economist, Dr. Eli Ginzberg (Ginzberg, 1991) reports that the significantly high birthrates of Mexican Americans indicate a greater need for access to prenatal and postnatal care for women and children. For Latinos/as on both sides of the U.S.–Mexico border, water and air pollution and the dumping of toxic waste threaten their health status. Recent reports show that California's Latino/a population has an incidence rate two to four times higher than non-Latino/a Caucasians for many sexually transmitted diseases, such as gonorrhea, chlamydia, and syphilis. These differences are higher in rural counties with a higher farmworker population (Latino Health News, 1994).

The health care needs identified thus far suggest that U.S. Latinos/as are ill served by current health care delivery systems, yet the definition of U.S. Latino/a community needs is inherently difficult. The difficulty lies within the reality that Latino/a people consist of subsets of different ethnic, racial, and larger groups. For example, migrant agricultural workers, immigrants, undocumented workers, resident aliens, and disenfranchised U.S. citizens are not all Latinos/as. However, many are; they come from varied Latino/a national origins and reside in different parts of the continental United States and Puerto Rico. The following section addresses some of these differences by reviewing the epidemiology of Latinos/as in Puerto Rico and the United States with particular attention to subgroups in New York, California, and Texas.

Subgroup Issues

Readers are reminded that the use of Latino/a or Hispanic as a descriptor is a statistically vague category, and can give rise to misleadingly inclusive portraits of Latinos/as or Hispanics having similar needs and access issues. Specific subgroup health disparities may differ due to one having a larger number of uninsured persons, another having greater linguistic barriers, and still another having more health problems (Schur, Bernstein, & Berk, 1987). Illustrative is the frequent report that Latinos/as are younger than the U.S. general population. However, it is Puerto Rican and Mexican descent Latinos/as who have a larger percent of people under 19 years old than does the total population. Latinos/as also are often described as primarily living in the 16 largest U.S. cities, yet Cubans are not concentrated in these cities and 41% of Mexicans reside in small cities and rural areas. Therefore, it is extremely important both to consider the loss of information that occurs when Latinos/as are grouped into homogeneous categories and to use specific information regarding the characteristics, behaviors, beliefs, attitudes, and knowledge of the culturally distinct individual Latino/a groups of Indigenous, Asian, European, or African descent to develop health and human services delivery systems responsive to their unique needs.

For example, the Latino/a poverty rate in the Northeast was 36.6% in 1987 and 23% in the West, yet Puerto Ricans on the continental U.S. had the highest poverty rate of any Latino/a subgroup (Center on Budget and Policy Priorities, 1988). New York City's Puerto Rican population of approximately 900,000 constituted 50% of the city's Latino/a population in 1990, yet they comprise only 12% of the national Latino/a population. Dominicans are the second largest group of Latino/a New Yorkers, with over 350,000 people (New York City Planning Commission [NYCPC], 1993). In 1990, 95% of New York City's homeless were Puerto Ricans and African Americans, with an additional estimated 50,000 Latino/a families living doubled and tripled up in crowded apartments (Nicot & Colon, 1990). The majority of Puerto Rican New Yorkers in 1990 were second-generation individuals born on the mainland (NYCPC, 1993).

The March 1993 Current Population Survey, conducted by the U.S. Census Bureau, estimated the labor force participation rate of Puerto Rican males 16 years of age or over to be 68.6%, yet total Latino males' average participation was 79.2%. Unemployment rates for all Latino males 16 years of age or more were estimated at 12.4%, yet Puerto Rican males' actually had a 17.2% rate. Poverty rates for Puerto Rican families in 1992 were estimated at 32.5%, while the Latino/a family average was 26.2 per cent (Institute for Puerto Rican Policy [IPRP], 1994). During the 1992–93 school year 36% of all New York City public school students were Latino/a, with 55% attending state designated low performing schools, 40% in vocational high schools, and 32% in academic high schools. Forty-one percent of all dropouts were Latino/a and 28% of Latino/a students were classified as having limited English proficiency (Nieves, 1994).

Excluding Puerto Rico, Puerto Ricans have a 37% poverty rate in the United States, as compared to 30% for Mexican Americans, 27% for Central and South Americans, 18% for Cuban Americans and 10% for non-Latino/a Caucasians. The rate for Puerto Rican single-female headed households is 60%, as compared to 25% for non-Latina Caucasians. In 1989, Puerto Rico had an overall poverty rate of 55% and a rate of 70% for single-female headed households. 1991 Aid to Families with Dependent Children (AFDC) data on people receiving welfare in the United States indicates 18% are Latinos/as, while they comprise 9% of the total U.S. population. In New York City, the 1990 census reports 35% of Puerto Rican households receiving public assistance compared to 13% of the total population. While in 1989, 31% of all households in Puerto Rico reported public assistance (Council on Scientific Affairs, 1991).

These figures provide important information to assess demographic determinants of need for Puerto Ricans; yet such data is not readily available for all Latino/a subgroups given the failure of federal and state governments to collect subgroup and gender-specific health and human service data. Existing literature focuses on Mexicans, Puerto Ricans, and Cubans, with scarce information on Central and South Americans, the fastest-growing subgroups among Latin Americans (Herrell, 1994). In part, this is related to a paucity of Latino/a administrators and policymakers in the health and human services bureaucracies. However, among the major reasons for the virtual nonexistence of data on Latino/a subgroups are: the exclusion of Latinos/as from one third of the 21 key Department of Health and Human Services (DHHS) data collection systems; the compromising of available data because of the elapsed time since the data was gathered; methodological failures in capturing geographic differences and rapid demographic changes; and the lack of data on major disease incidence by gender in Latino/a subgroups (Valdez, et al., 1992).

Advocacy Positions

Based on the health care and human service needs stated above, and access problems faced by the Latino/a community, policy researchers and advocates have suggested that comprehensive health planning for Latinos/as should include mental health, substance abuse, long-term care and residential services, community outreach, case management, and health education services (Carrillo, 1993). Also advocated are human services in community based and family settings, including home care, early intervention, and unified systems of care in schools and workplaces as part and parcel of comprehensive planning (Center for Health Policy Development [CHPD], 1993).

The Texas-based Center for Health Policy Development (Ortiz, 1993) calls for proactive family and community health models including maternal-infant care, immunization, nutrition, and elder care. It also advocates environmental and occupational health services targeting at-risk children, female adolescents, men from 13 to 40 years old, and the health needs of mobile populations, i.e., migrants, refugees, farmworkers, and immigrants. The Center's view of a quality service delivery system includes health promotion and disease prevention initiatives in recreation centers, public housing projects, community colleges (which have the largest concentration of Latinos/as in higher education), and correctional settings (i.e., youth incarceration centers, jails, prisons, halfway houses).

The National Congress for Puerto Rican Rights argues for culturally competent care for all Latinos/as and residents of the United States (including those in Puerto Rico) and inclusion of a comprehensive "healthy living" education campaign as an integral part of any basic health plan (Latino Coalition for a Healthy California [LCHC], 1994a). West Coast Latinos/as have similarly argued that without such consumer education and orientation in place, Latinos/as may not fully enjoy the benefits of comprehensive health coverage (LCHC, 1993). The Latino Coalition for a Healthy California (LCHC, 1994a) advocates for providing comprehensive health care to the undocumented in community non-profit clinics, county and local public health departments, and migrant and rural health centers. These historically underfunded "safety net" providers are already providing services to this population and typically do not refuse service on the basis of legal status or national origin. Since Latino/a families may have members who are undocumented, comprehensive family health planning must include these individuals. At a minimum, based on reasonable medical standards, the services offered to the undocumented should include clinical preventive services, communicable diseases, emergency and ambulatory medical and surgical services, family planning services and services for pregnant women, pediatric care and primary care (LCHC, 1994a)

While opponents will argue the fiscal burden of providing and reimbursing care to the undocumented, the homeless and transients, the long term medical, financial, and public health impact of inattention to these populations will be more costly as the failure to provide early diagnosis and treatment of communicable diseases poses greater risks to the health of the public at large (LCHC, 1994a). One solution suggests inclusion of multidisciplinary health care providers such as mental health workers, health promoters, paraprofessionals, and outreach workers (Perez, 1994) in the service delivery system. Another would stress the importance of culturally competent programming to include the availability of health care prevention materials in the language of the target populations and the relevance of these materials to Latinos/as' beliefs regarding their health conditions.

As one of the nation's largest safety-net providers to underserved Latino/a communities, the New York City Health and Hospitals Corporation (HHC) is building networks to provide a comprehensive array of services and continuum of care, i.e., preventive, primary, specialty, hospital, and long-term care. HHC has advocated for the reduction or elimination of co-payments in suggested health reform plans in recognition of the fact that co-payments of $5 to $25 dollars are clearly not considered small or modest for poor and special needs populations (New York City Health and Hospitals Corporation [NYCHHC], 1994e). These payments cause hardship for many, deter many from seeking timely, appropriate care, and create administrative burdens for safety-net providers in their attempts at fee collection. HHC also recognizes the need for enhanced services to poor and vulnerable populations, such as social services, transportation, translation, and interpreter services.

A final advocacy position is that health coverage for migrant farmworkers must be portable. They are a mobile population that works seasonally for numerous and varied employers throughout the individual states of the nation. Health coverage must be available where their jobs are, and when they need it. Currently, region-alized managed care and managed competition plans do not include portability, leading many advocates to argue for a nation-wide universal coverage system that provides primary, preventive, urgent, and emergency care to overcome geographic barriers to health services (California Rural Legal Assistance, 1994).

YIN-YANG:
HEALTHY BALANCE WITH ASIAN COMMUNITIES

As in the earlier section, issues for the Asian community have parallels in other communities of color. They are described separately for Asian Americans in order to preserve the uniqueness of issues and needs. For Asians in their countries of origin, the balance of yin-yang qualities is considered critical to good health and well being. Basic essences of the body include: Qi (wind), blood, and yin and yang qualities. These qualities represent the balance between hot and cold, male and female elements which must be kept in balance to remain healthy. They are followed by pathologic factors of wind, moisture, and toxins which cause illness. Deficiencies of yin will give rise to symptoms of dryness (e.g., dry mouth, cough) and heat (e.g., fever, inflammation) while deficiencies of yang give rise to symptoms of poor vitality and strength (e.g., fatigue, impotence), and lack of adequate warmth (e.g., chills). Deficiencies are caused by the failure of one to regulate the other (i.e., yin-yang balance). In looking at health care needs of Asian Americans, we need to recognize the importance of this balance in weighing choice of providers, utilization patterns, medical compliance, and evaluating service delivery systems. More important, these views carry themselves beyond the practices of immigrant/refugee populations.

Health Status and Needs

For many, the myth of a model minority suggests that Asian Americans are healthy, wealthy, and wise. The Asian Pacific Islander American population has been the fastest growing population in the United States for over two decades. By the year 2000, they are expected to make up almost 11% of the total population. The 1990 Census shows that the Asian population in the United States grew from 1.7 million in 1970 to 7.3 million in 1990. Despite this marked growth in population, documentation of health status of Asian Americans is seriously lacking. While public health statistics generally

show that Asian Americans demonstrate better health status compared to Caucasians and other groups of color, failure to desegregate
Asian groups and their small sample size in most studies result in
misleading data on Asian American health status. The paucity of
data and the ethnocultural barriers to care have been well docu-
mented (Lin-Fu, 1993). This was most marked in the Secretary's Task
Force Report on Minority Health in 1985, which failed to show disparities among Asian Americans and declared Asian Americans a
healthy minority. Omitted from the discussion was the small size of
the Asian American samples, and the selection of mortality indicators less relevant to Asian American groups. In fact, disparities in
health status on hepatitis B and tuberculosis among Asian Americans
are apparent with rates that exceed 10 times that among Caucasian
communities when methodological issues are corrected (South Cove
Community Health Center [SCCHC], 1994). In an overview of
methodological issues (Yu & Liu, 1994), Yu points out that our
knowledge of Asian American health status is, in fact, based on only
a few epidemiological surveys conducted, generally, in Hawaii or
California, and on inferences drawn from data of the National Center
for Health Statistics. Moreover, these data typically do not sample
new immigrants and refugees. Numerous methodological problems
include: how the study population is defined, inadequate sampling
of rare elements, developing instruments that need to be translated,
determining actual response rates, and obtaining informed consent.

Health status and service needs of the Asian American community are distinct from that of the general population (Chin, 1991).
The prevalence of active tuberculosis is about 310 per 100,000
among Southeast Asians, 40.5 per 100,000 among all Asians, and
only 4 per 100,000 among Caucasians. Eighty percent of newly arrived Asian immigrants and refugees usually carry parasitic disease
infection. Giardia and amebiasis show an 18% and 40% rate respectively, compared to 4% and 3% in the general population respectively. Fifty-five percent of malaria cases in the United States occur
among Southeast Asian refugees. Seventeen percent of Asian Americans compared with 1% in the general population are chronic
hepatitis B carriers. In 1987, Asian Americans had the highest morbidity rate of hepatitis infection of any group in the United States.
Asian Americans are more frequently diagnosed with hepatoma,
lung and nasopharyngeal carcinomas possibly due to a higher incidence (70%) of smoking among Asian American males compared to
the incidence (25%) in the general population. Sixteen percent of
mental health service users carry a diagnosis of depression; 22% of
mental health service users carry a diagnosis of psychosis. Suicide is

higher among a student population for reasons associated with academic achievement, while it is also higher for Chinese American women over 40. While the prevalence of HIV/AIDS in the Asian community is low, rates of growth identified in New York City show that it tripled over a three year period (SCCHC, 1994).

Given the diversity within the Asian population, and the fact that greater than 50% of Asian Americans in the United States are immigrants and refugees, language and cultural factors play a significant rote in influencing access to health care utilization (Mayeno & Hirola, 1990). The seriousness of these barriers in accessing health care is compounded by poverty, lack of data documenting the need within specific ethnic groups, and institutional policies which mitigate against culturally competent care. The high rate of uninsured (only 53% of Asian Americans have employment based health insurance compared to 69% of non-Latino/a Caucasians), and the low annual rate of physician visits per person (four per person versus six per person for Caucasians) illustrate these problems of access.

Important among the health needs of Asian Americans is the common use of herbal medicine and traditional Asian methods of health care in combination with Western health care methods. The U.S. health care system has not accepted these methods as valid when evaluating compliance or as eligible for reimbursement.

Subgroup Issues

With over 30 different Asian subgroups in the United States, the importance of understanding health care needs of specific ethnic groups is imperative, especially when the failure to desegregate data on Asian Americans has led to a masking of their specific health needs and misinterpretations because of bipolar distribution within many ethnic groups (Takeuchi & Young, 1990). While documenting the health needs of specific ethnic groups goes beyond the scope of this book, sources exist which document health issues of Korean Americans (Koh & Koh, 1993), of Pacific Americans (Chen, 1994),of Chinese Americans (Chen, 1995), and of Asian Americans in general (Zane, Takeuchi, & Young, 1994).

Advocacy Positions

Three national organizations have advocated for Asian American health and mental health needs and issues. The Association of Asian Pacific Community Health Organization (AAPCHO), National Asian Pacific American Families Against Substance Abuse (NAPAFASA), and Asian Pacific Islander American Health Forum (APIAHF) have formed networks of community-based agencies and professionals toward creating policy and practice which further the health care needs of Asian American communities. Policy papers (Association of Asian Pacific Community Health Organizations [AAPCHO], 1993; Forman, Lu, Leung, & Ponce, 1990) outline access problems, and fact sheets (Asian American Health Forum, 1990) outline various risk factors and diseases that vividly display the disparities in health status for specific Asian Pacific Islander (API) subgroups. Most important, these organizations have advocated for principles of cultural competence, linguistic appropriateness, and community-based care under any system of care with an attention to specific ethnic groups. The need for health education, community outreach, and care management to ensure quality and competent services is underscored. While these positions are generally accepted by policymakers and legislators, there has been a failure to provide the resources or infrastructures to achieve successful outcomes. For example, Healthy People 2000, a broad based federal initiative released in 1990 to improve the health of all people through an emphasis on the prevention of health problems, failed to include significant objectives targeting Asian Americans. Although its overt objective was to aim specifically at groups who bear a disproportionate share of disease, disability, and premature death compared to the general population, it fell short of this mark. Second, the Disadvantaged Minority Health Improvement Act of 1990, intended to improve health care access for communities of color, authorized the Office of Minority Health to provide assistance to primary and preventive health care entities in the provision of bilingual/bicultural services; yet, only $3 million was appropriated for the country for one year to ensure linguistic-appropriate services.

FROM TRAUMA TO WELLNESS: SOCIETAL HEALTH WITHIN AFRICAN AMERICAN COMMUNITIES

African Americans have a proud but traumatic history in the United States. Adversities that began with slavery and currently include racism, discrimination, and prejudice have had a significant impact on the present health status of this population. These adversities have also made it difficult for many African Americans to re-conceptualize the goal of healthy minds, bodies, and communities (Davis & Jordan, 1994). Although the oppression this group has endured bears some similarity to that of other oppressed groups in the United States, it has been both severe and intractable. Over years the oppression of African Americans has been exhibited by:

- a systematic cutoff from folk and ethnomedical approaches to health care
- denial of access to traditional health care for more than a century
- substandard health care and health education intergenerationally
- the devaluation of group characteristics (i.e., cognitive, biological, interpersonal) by the dominant culture and the internalization of these misperceptions by some African Americans
- a history of being rewarded for service to/caretaking of the dominant culture rather than self-care taking
- subjection to deep psychological pain that, in some instances, has compromised the ability to feel and therefore the capacity to express love and affection (hooks, 1994)
- systematic and persistent threats to the well-being of the group that have forced a preoccupation with immediate/basic survival rather than lasting prosperity
- alienation and marginalization by the dominant culture
- the reality that for some youths a sense of belonging is based on a bond of risky and destructive behavior which develops into a way of life (e.g., substance abuse, gang violence) (Cummings & DeHart, 1995)

Indeed, the historical societal status of African Americans has endowed many with remarkable strengths. Yet, in many instances this has also nurtured the development of self-defeating attitudes, beliefs, and practices (e.g., improper diet, long hours of work with little rest, inadequate attention to general health needs, ambivalence about self-care including asking for help when appropriate) which continue to take a toll on the overall health and well-being of this population. Despite these challenges there are hopeful signs that African Americans have started to take a proactive stance on health issues. Much remains to be done, however, for many within this population to achieve wellness.

Health Status and Needs

In an analysis of implications of health care reform for African Americans, Washington (Washington, 1995) contends that comparisons of various measures of African American health to that of their Caucasian counterparts appear as if they are ". . . between groups in two different countries, a sort of medical apartheid." This duality is manifested by the sobering realities that African Americans ". . . are screened for illnesses less often, get sick more frequently, are diagnosed later, are treated less aggressively, and are buried earlier than whites" (p. 34).

The Task Force on Minority Health (U.S. Department of Health and Human Services [USDHHS], 1985) indicates that African Americans show a 1.5% greater likelihood of succumbing to major causes of death than Caucasians. Heart disease is the number one killer of African Americans. Between 1985 and 1992, the rate of AIDS and HIV infection increased by 26% for this population. In addition, hypertension, cardiovascular disease, kidney disease, substance abuse, and related conditions (i.e., cirrhosis, hepatitis, diabetes, lung disease, some forms of cancer, and infant mortality) are particularly prevalent in African American communities even though these illnesses are highly preventable. The psychological stress associated with long term oppression is often related to the development, severity, and persistence of these conditions. Hypertension and diabetes are so common within this population that some African Americans speak of these illnesses as though contracting them is inevitable. Hypertension affects one in three African Americans while approximately three million (i.e., 1 in 10) have diabetes. Another recent and disturbing development is the increasing incidence of tuberculosis in this population. This disease, which was under control for many years, rose by 26% between 1985 and 1992. It is also disturbing that many African Americans live in areas where toxic wastes are dumped or emitted into the air. Such pollution increases the vulnerability of these residents to some forms of cancer, miscarriage, and birth defects, asthma and other respiratory illnesses.

The ratio of African American women to Caucasian women who succumb to the major causes of death is more than 4:1; the average African American woman dies 5.5 years earlier than her white counterpart. The leading cause of death for African American men is lung cancer while the incidence of prostate cancer is 40% higher for this group than for Caucasian men. In 1991, the life expectancy for African American men was 65.6 as compared to 73.4 years for Caucasian men, while the ratio of African American men to Caucasian men for death by homicide alone was 6:1.

AIDS and HIV infection are taking an enormous toll on African American communities. Even though members of this group account for only 12% of the population of the United States, 30% of those who have contracted AIDS have been African American. HIV rates for African Americans increased 19% between 1990 and 1992 and AIDS has become the leading cause of death for black men between the ages of 25 and 44, according to the most recent reports from the Centers for Disease Control (U.S. Bureau of the Census, 1993). At the end of 1993, the reported number of AIDS cases among African American women exceeded 25,000 (Coleman, 1996). Fifty-three percent of women and adolescents with the AIDS virus reported in 1993 were African Americans (Smith, 1995). It is also believed that more recently the majority of women and children infected with the HIV virus are African American. In view of the probability that this illness is still under-reported, the actual figure for women who contract HIV infection is probably higher. While African Americans are over-represented in nearly every HIV risk group (Centers for Disease Control, 1993), estimates indicate that approximately one-third of African American women take no preventative measures against the risk of this infection (U.S. Bureau of the Census, 1993; Jemmott & Jemmott, 1991).

There are many other significant threats to the health of African-American women. In addition to incidences of sexually transmitted diseases and pelvic inflammatory disease within this population, cigarette smoking and deaths due to breast cancer, cervical cancer, and earlier onset heart disease frequently occur. Breast cancer is the leading cause of death in African American women, while cervical cancer strikes this population three times more often than Caucasian women. Furthermore, African American women are twice as likely as their white counterparts to die from this disease (Mays & Cohran, 1988). Fibroid tumors of the uterus is a condition that affects 40% of African American women between the late twenties and mid-forties. Between 50 and 75% of this population has a chance of developing this condition, which is often intergenerational (Villarosa, 1994). Fibroids are thought to be linked to poor nutrition (i.e., diet high in fat and cholesterol content), high stress levels, and other lifestyle issues. Although this condition is not life threatening, it commonly causes significant difficulties (i.e., pain and discomfort, anemia, fertility problems) in 50% of those African American women who develop them. Prior to the use of modern medical procedures (i.e., laser surgery, myomectomy) and awareness of the value of holistic health strategies (i.e., meditation, yoga, regular exercise, herbal medicine), many African American women of childbearing age had hysterectomies as a result of this condition.

Another particularly disturbing reality associated with the reproductive health of African American women is that fewer are likely to have early prenatal care than Caucasian women even though African American women are less likely to have abortions. Lack of prenatal care, and smoking during pregnancy are related to development of fetal alcohol syndrome and infants born addicted to crack cocaine in inner-city African American communities. Many of these infants die within the first year of life and account for the 2:1 ratio of infant mortality for African Americans compared to that for Caucasians (Villarosa, 1994).

The societal health status of African American men is particularly disturbing. Majors and Billson (Majors & Billson, 1992) contend that this population has the highest rate of important indicators of social stress in the United States with the exception of Native American men. They associate this with the rise in mental disorders, intra-group homicide and other forms of criminal behavior (e.g., domestic violence, substance abuse), and incarceration rates which are disproportionately high for this population. An emphasis on health care delivery to the entire family unit could become one means of addressing the health care needs of African American men more effectively. Presently, this population is marginalized by a focus on the needs of women and children.

The fact that a disproportionate number of African Americans are uninsured poses a major obstacle to their ability to access preventive, timely, and quality health care as opposed to inadequate but expensive care in hospital emergency rooms, and expensive radical treatment for advanced diseases. African Americans constitute at least 21.9 percent of the 37 million United States citizens under the age of 65 who are uninsured with no resources, while Caucasians constitute 14.5 percent of this population. The Clinton administration proposes that true universal coverage is the solution for improving the health status of African Americans. Yet, Washington reminds us that ". . . major groups with large constituencies of African Americans—the poor, small business owners, prisoners and undocumented residents of the United States—are excluded from the universal coverage that the Clinton administration's plan [for] health reform has promised . . . financial supports needed by the poor have been underestimated" (p. 34).

Despite the reality that some of the problems that beset African American communities seem to be nearing genocidal proportions, attention to prevention and wellness is stronger than ever before. Yet, in view of the health status of this group, obviously much remains to be done to improve its plight. Positive attention to prevention and wellness is reflected in the increasing availability of literature on African American health issues that is targeted for lay persons; much of this literature stresses the mind-body-spiritual connection and prevention. Also prominent are endeavors of the National Black Women's Health Project (Atlanta), the Institute on Black Chemical Abuse, the Black Men's Campaign on AIDS (Boston), the National Association of Black Psychologists' workshops on AIDS and HIV infection, sponsorship of community health and wellness fairs by prominent African American organizations, and the creation of ethnoculture-specific initiatives by community health centers. Furthermore, the number of African American health and mental health professionals is also increasing even though this population is still considerably disproportionate to the actual size and needs of the African American population.

Advocacy

Clearly, universal health coverage is needed if the overall health status of the African American population is to improve at a significant level. In addition, research is needed to assess the ongoing health-related education needs of African American communities. Particular attention must be paid to eradicating social and environmental conditions that compromise the health and well-being of this population. Furthermore, more attention to high incidence illnesses is needed. In addition, the identification of life practices that contribute to wellness as well as the onset of illness and untimely death is needed to facilitate early case finding, prevention, effective treatment, and follow-up care. The systematic inclusion of consumer input on policy and practice issues would encourage more African Americans to take a proactive stance.

CROSSCUTTING HEALTH CARE NEEDS

While coming from different perspectives, communities of color face some common issues and problems in meeting their health care needs. Though common solutions to similar access problems bond our communities together, we must underscore the importance of respecting the unique and diverse ways our communities have arrived at these solutions. The following list attempts to identify these crosscutting health care access problems/issues in communities of color. Without the earlier discussion, the issues listed would perhaps appear overly simplistic or insignificant.

Policy

- Lack of persons of color in health care management and policy positions resulting in failures to understand unique needs
- Failure to include persons of color to participate in Request For Proposal development and review to ensure cultural competency of health service programs

- Lack of coordinated lobbying on behalf of communities of color
- Community-based organizations serving communities of color lack access to U.S. Public Health Service policymakers
- Regulations based on geography frequently neglect population needs, thereby excluding migrant/seasonal farmworkers, children, homeless people, rural residents, immigrants, and refugees from health care service delivery systems
- Emphasis in health care fails to include environmental issues
- Communities of color are often subsumed and neglected under the label of "minority" in federal, state, local, public, and private health planning

Reimbursement

- Lack of health insurance; employment often does not include it as a benefit because of piecework wages
- Restrictions in eligibility criteria for Medicaid coverage, i.e., migrant workers, immigrant status
- Non-reimbursement for primary and preventive health care services, or for "alternative" healing practices

Training

- Lack of cultural competency training in the training of health professionals, resulting in inappropriate methods for treating communities of color
- Limited pool of bilingual-bicultural providers to deliver services

Research/Data

- Lack of relevant research identifying health care delivery needs and strategies which promote health care access, utilization, and effectiveness for communities of color
- Racial, ethnic, gender, and language diversity is often ignored when communities of color are lumped together under the label of "minority," "Hispanic," "Black," or "Asian" in health care planning

Service Delivery

- Lack of child care, transportation, weekend and evening clinics given lower use of babysitters, and inability to get paid release time from work for medical care

- Few economic incentives for health providers to serve low income populations and communities of color
- Poor access to prenatal care because of language and cultural barriers
- Public health initiatives, health promotion, and community education not available in languages other than English or relevant to the health beliefs of communities of color
- Lack of health care facilities providing culturally competent services to communities of color
- Inadequate linkages between private providers, local health departments, and community health centers
- Delayed entry into primary and preventive care because of access problems results in overutilization of emergency services
- Lack of innovative expansion in "nontraditional methods" in providing care (i.e., nurse practitioners, dental hygienists, health psychologists, international medical or health service graduates, physician assistants)
- Inadequate social and health services to assist successful reentry into the community i.e., released prisoners, persons discharged from psychiatric hospitals

In summary, health research findings indicate that a multiservice, community informed practice is critical to meeting health care and human service needs of subpopulations among communities of color. Current health care delivery systems serving these subgroups are grossly inadequate. Furthermore, problem definition is a complex task due to the vast diversity among Latinos/as, Asian Americans, and African Americans. Therefore, advocacy for these subgroups must be comprehensive and inclusive of clinical, health education, and community services. A universal coverage system might eradicate geographic barriers to service especially if the emphasis is on universal access to ensure inclusion of all segments of the population.

COMMENTARY

G. Rita Dudley Grant

In Chapter One an important statement is made for all health care professionals, providers, researchers, and most importantly policy makers regarding the necessity of including cultural and subcultural indices in health care delivery systems. Of great significance is the psychological import of these observations. Health has been identified as a right and goal that is aspired to for all U.S. citizens by C. Everett Koop, M.D., former Surgeon General in his Healthy People 2000 program for the country. Moreover, it has been increasingly recognized that the health of any individual is directly connected to his or her psychological state. Disease prevention and recovery can ultimately be seen to reflect the emotional health of the individual (Matarazzo, 1984). When considering the broader perspective, it can also be seen to reflect the psychosocial/emotional health of any given community.

In Chapter One, the authors reflect on the community needs of each of the three cultural groups under consideration, Latinos/as, Asian Americans, and African Americans. In each instance, the demographics are alarming. Latinos/as are more at risk for a host of illnesses, while lacking access to health care to prevent the development of these diseases. Many from this population fall into the further disenfranchised subgroups of immigrants or migrant workers with little or no access or right to health care delivery. The point is made that policymakers must consider subgroup needs if adequate health care is to be provided to these very at-risk groups. Asian Americans too, have their share of access difficulties. Immigration is also a problem for this population, as is the problem of culturally consonant access. The myth of the model minority, belies needs poignantly detailed in the chapter. Thus, the Asian population is overlooked when thought is given to designing programs which attempt to reach out to minority communities.

Perhaps the population which has been studied the most in terms of lack of access is the African American community. Chronically underserved, with the issue of intentional or unconscious genocide always "lurking in the background," the statistics clearly show that comprehensive health care delivery for this population has not truly been addressed by policymakers. Rather, the indices associated with the health status of this population reflect a systematic decline in the health of the population. Infant mortality is increasing rather than decreasing, despite the excellent research and information disseminated by Rowley et al (1993) of the Centers for Disease Control regarding risk factors and recommendations for mitigation of the enormous infant mortality rate in the inner city black community.

A recent issue of the American Psychologist (APA, 1997) was devoted to psychology and public health. In the lead article on women's health, the authors acknowledge that stressful life events are linked to a modest increase in risk for a variety of chronic diseases as well as an increase in recurrent health problems in those already suffering from disease; and that such events can alter the effectiveness of treatment (Matthews et al, 1997). These authors also make the point that in their planned women's study of health issues, a concerted effort was made to include women of diverse ethnicity. However, it was acknowledged that most of the scales utilized had not previously been standardized on these populations.

A troubling consideration in the lack of adequate health care for ethnic minorities is the issue of responsibility. There is a dearth of diverse health professionals to provide culturally consonant health care. Thus, issues of training become paramount, not only in the expansion of the pool of minority providers, but in the increase of sensitivity among all providers to the special needs of these populations.

This chapter then, dramatically and in a detailed manner, puts forth the plight of ethnic minority health care delivery, and the need for expansion, consideration, and change in the current delivery system. Crosscutting issues generate considerable concern regarding the possibility of addressing these wide-ranging issues from advocacy and policy to training and service delivery. Perhaps the greatest challenge to the behavioral health professional is the creation of strategies to disseminate this information to public policy makers and the public at large. Recognizing the gaps is the first step, albeit a crucial one, in bringing about change in the health status of ethnic minorities. This chapter can be seen as a call to action. We must be willing to become active in public policy arenas, continue to research more effective alternatives for health care delivery, and ensure the dissemination of the information to those who can make a difference. The authors have outlined the issues well. It is now the responsibility of all behavioral health scientists/practitioners and those committed to equity in health care to respond to these issues and the inherent challenge to create health for all.

2

Strategies and Mechanisms for Meeting the Health Care Needs of Communities of Color

Victor De La Cancela,
Jean Lau Chin, and Yvonne M. Jenkins

In the previous chapter, we identified the diverse health needs of people of color, and suggested that the inability of sociopolitical and health care systems to competently respond to cultural and community differences results in decreased access to and acceptability of health care systems among the poor and biopsychosocially underserved. We suggested community health psychology as an approach to attend to those psychocultural factors which clinical health psychology within the United States has ignored. In this chapter, we shift our focus to consideration of health systems reform and provide recommendations for how health care services within an ideal program can meet those needs specific to Latino/a, Asian, and African American groups. We provide a broad overview of community health promotion and disease prevention as a holistic and comprehensive approach. Interventions in the areas of substance use, AIDS/HIV and violence are provided as examples of public health problems with psychological consequences that disproportionately affect disenfranchised communities of color.

Much of what we describe as strategies and mechanisms have public policy implications and suggest advocacy positions needed to effect change in order to promote community empowerment and cultural competence. They are relevant to all communities of color as a community oriented approach to health psychology. However, differences between different communities of color continue to be stressed to avoid dilution of those specific needs communities of color face, and the potential danger of presuming that all needs can be met through a singular model. Thus, unique examples for Latinos/as, Asian Americans, and African Americans will be provided along with cross-cutting issues and principles.

HEALTH SYSTEMS REFORM

Some issues for health systems reform remain the same while their manifestations within communities differ. The high incidence of uninsureds in Asian communities often results from the high number of workers employed in piecework jobs or jobs without health benefits, i.e., garment and restaurant workers, yet the same problem in Latino/a communities results from the high number of migrant workers, i.e., farmworkers. However, the problem faced by both groups is the inability to access linguistically appropriate and culturally competent services. Ideally, systems of care for communities of color would ensure universal access, comprehensive services, universal coverage, and cultural competence. They would include explicitly defined benefits and coverage which are relevant to that community for primary, acute, chronic, developmental, and long-term care; they would not discriminate among segments of the communities through deductibles or coinsurance for legal immigrants, undocumented individuals, part-time, seasonal, and temporary workers or their dependents. Coverage would also be portable. While public policy opponents would argue the costliness of such an ideal program, it is our contention that a truly culturally competent system would, in fact, be more cost effective because it avoids pitfalls in the current system which treat communities of color as secondary or "special" populations in the provision of care. Such a program would avoid duplication of effort resulting from lack of culturally relevant diagnosis and treatment, untimely delays due to unavailable or poorly trained interpreters, and poor risk management due to inappropriate use of medical interventions for specific populations.

AN IDEAL HEALTH CARE SERVICES PROGRAM

An ideal health care services program would include those elements which are relevant to the health beliefs and practices of specific communities, responsive to the health risks prevalent in those communities, and flexible enough to meet the unique needs of diverse groups. These elements would be comprehensive and provide continuity from preventive, primary, and tertiary care systems. Barriers such as copayments or noncoverage of special needs relevant to specific communities would not exist. Services would be linguistically appropriate with providers able to communicate in the patient's primary language. Families would also be involved in the planning of services, in the development and management of individualized treatment plans, and in the delivery and coordination of multiple services, reflecting an ecological and family-oriented approach to care. Ultimately, it would meet public health objectives in promoting the health of communities. An outline of these characteristics follows:

Primary and Preventive Care

- Vision care
- Hearing care
- Dental care, including preventive, diagnostic, and emergency services without any copayment, with broad coverage for those with special needs, covering dentures for adults, and interceptive orthodontics for children
- Health education counseling and classes in patients' primary language, relevant to health risks faced by their specific community
- Nutrition education counseling and classes
- Coverage of prescription drugs, including herbal medicines
- Mental health services including outpatient treatment promoting the linkage of such services with primary and preventive health care services
- Behavioral health services including biofeedback, stress management, and smoking cessation
- Preventive services for children and adults, including immunizations and periodic screening, without cost sharing
- Pregnancy-related services, with abortion services and counseling
- Family planning services
- Transitional services from prison to community
- Coverage of preventive services where specific risks are high, i.e., hepatitis B vaccination for Asian population

Acute Care

- Emergency services, including ambulance
- Lab and diagnostic services
- Unlimited hospital care

Chronic/Long-Term Care

- Mental health and substance abuse benefits, including intensive residential and community-based care, and in-patient hospital services that achieve parity with medical hospital services
- Long-term care using a community-based model, including case management, adult day health care, hospice, home health care, extended nursing care
- Home dialysis
- Occupational health, rehabilitation, and habilitation services
- Durable medical equipment
- Prosthetic and orthopedic devices

Enabling Services

- Transportation for health care visits for those without cars
- Accommodations for family members in health care facilities to promote family-oriented care
- Evening and weekend service hours to accommodate the schedules of workers without paid leave for medical visits
- Mobile services in hard-to-reach sites and populations
- Translation services at all points of patient contact

As an *ideal* program, this is an example of the comprehensive coverage that can be fashioned for communities of color attending to the range of their priority biopsychosocial needs. It explicitly allows the services of certified and state licensed health service providers such as clinical psychologists and health educators that a more medically oriented model might omit. It also includes enabling services needed to promote access to care. This program builds on the advocacy to promote access and reduce barriers to care conducted by such groups as the Latino Coalition for a Healthy California (LCHC, 1992), Association of Asian Pacific Community Health Organizations (AAPCHO) (AAPCHO, 1993), and the body of opinion extant in the research literature about culturally competent care. Consequently, it serves as a yardstick by which communities of color and other medically underserved populations can measure the comprehensiveness and competency of services as service delivery systems undergo health care reform.

Vital to the principle of universal access is the inclusion of groups such as undocumented residents, a factor which is likely to give rise to criticism and controversy. However, the exclusion of these groups ignores the fact that many undocumented residents are also taxpayers supporting the U.S. economy through taxes on their salaries and on their purchases (LCHC, 1994b). Given that their tax dollars support programs denied to them, their exclusion raises the issue of human and civil rights violations. As federal and state laws mandate the provision of essential services to all residents regardless of immigration status, a position supported by the Latino Coalition for a Healthy California in their adoption of the doctrine of presumptive eligibility, such exclusion reflects a failure of cultural competence.

Finally, this policy position is also cost effective because it avoids more costly tertiary care and emergency room usage when primary and preventive care services are denied or made inaccessible. It is consistent with federal law, which provides emergency care and services necessary for the treatment of emergency medical conditions, and medically necessary services related to pregnancy, including prenatal care for undocumented residents. It is also consistent with medical ethics and federal and state laws that explicitly prohibit doctors and hospitals from turning away women in labor whatever their immigration status (LCHC, 1994b).

COMMUNITY-ORIENTED SERVICES

The health care programs, services, policies, and advocacy already described share an emphasis on primary and preventive care, universal access, and community-oriented service delivery. These characteristics need to be included when strategies are formed by community agencies operated by people of color. Community-oriented services involve collaboration among diverse agencies providing health, psychology, education, youth, and human services to communities of color. Partnerships between community agencies and "mainstream agencies" are needed with both shared and unique responsibilities. Agencies of color must further develop the community's organizational infrastructure while mainstream agencies must enhance their responsiveness to communities of color. Gone should be the days when agencies of color are marginalized as temporary layovers for clients unable to use mainstream services.

COMMUNITY EMPOWERMENT

Given our view of community health psychology as building healthy body, mind, and spirit for all peoples, strategies must build connections with communities of color, and provide the tools through which they can become empowered to get their needs met. These connections have been facilitated by the growing number of psychologists of color with a commitment to linguistic and cultural diversity, who have developed resources and outreach to communities of color. Applied fields of sociology, anthropology, and public health have also played a significant role with ethnocultural psychology in envisioning the total health of the larger community as a major concern, and in advocacy for community-oriented services that are truly autonomous and garnered by community strengths. These collaborations, community coalitions, and interorganizational planning have advantages for communities of color. For as boards of directors can be made more responsive by increased participation by persons of color, and as increased advocacy can influence policymakers, government staff, business/community leaders, and health service professionals, the development of community-oriented services can indeed be achieved.

Since the 1970s, many psychologists have engaged in community efforts and provided leadership to promote ethnoracial and cultural program development, increased outreach to communities of color, and heightened awareness of socioeconomic factors. Clinical-community psychologists in Latino/a, Asian American, and African American communities have become increasingly involved with job and literacy training, supportive housing, gang prevention, substance abuse prevention, homicide-related bereavement, child care, parent education, school-based counseling, correctional health support, and teenage pregnancy prevention; in essence, a wide range of health-related and prevention focus initiatives previously not defined as the domain of psychology. These roles have been a result of the increased recognition of the interrelatedness of biopsychosociocultural contexts to community, psychological, and physical well-being. They have consistently found that their effectiveness is dependent on community involvement and their responsiveness to community needs, community organization, community ownership, and priority setting. In fact, the essence of community-oriented services has been prevention, enrichment, and a holistic approach to health programming.

A HOLISTIC APPROACH

The strategy of a holistic approach at a community level, as opposed to its more usual application to individuals, is significant for community-oriented services. From this vantage point, communities of color develop connection and bonding among their members; we might call this culture or the interdependency inherent in our views of health and quality of life. Nevertheless, a holistic approach needs to respect and maintain those specific differences important to our communities. In the Asian immigrant community, for example, a holistic approach is reflected in service utilization where help-seeking behaviors of Asians tend to be generic, i.e., health providers are viewed as generic problem solvers, able to meet multiple and comprehensive needs ranging from health to social services. Consequently, case management and social services become an integral part of health care delivery for Asian Americans.

A holistic approach to health care planning and service delivery contradicts the past emphasis in health and mental health care on specialization. The separation of psychological and physical states has been reinforced by the historical separation between health and mental health as discrete service delivery systems. This discrete and specialized approach to health care is currently being questioned; its beneficiaries have been the specialists able to garner enhanced reimbursements. In fact, specialization and a discrete approach to health care have been irrelevant and insensitive to the ways in which communities of color, and perhaps people in general, think about their health. In essence, a holistic approach to health care planning will challenge existing concepts and practices in our health care system; it will challenge its basic organizational structures, underlying assumptions, and operating principles which have failed to meet the health needs of communities of color.

COLLABORATION

Among the strategies and mechanisms for meeting the health care needs of communities of color, collaboration, coalition building, and interorganizational planning are essential (Petrovich, 1987). Collaborative efforts must be increased among public, private, and community-based organizations to enhance cost-effective strategies for serving communities of color. Regional alliances for communities of color can be established to optimize economies of scale on administrative costs, supplies, and equipment as group purchasing arrangements for health insurance become more common. Consortia fundraising and joint ventures organized around regional areas or health needs specific to communities may enhance responsiveness from grantmakers as resources shrink. Service improvement can occur through interagency coordination. A shared agenda is needed among civic associations, higher education, police athletic leagues, religious agencies (e.g., Catholic charities), youth recreational clubs (Boys Clubs, YMCAs), and the philanthropic community if biopsychosociocultural contexts are to be integrated.

While community-based organizations must increasingly collaborate to survive and thrive in a new health care environment, mainstream organizations must also share in this responsibility. Corporations and local chambers of commerce can create greater community linkages and partnerships with communities of color. For example, they can develop leadership initiatives among youth of color, establish internships and training in fiscal management, provide corporate in-kind contributions and executive-on-loan programs, and support affordable housing. The private sector can support the establishment of a clearinghouse of successful community development programs which can be replicated in new settings. Collaboration with universities and public health agencies can provide data and research specific to ethnic, racial, and cultural subgroups for health care planning; dissemination of research data for lay audiences, communities, human service providers, legislators, and policymakers can be used to promote change (Herrell, 1994). Advocacy to promote change becomes one aspect of such collaboration.

PUBLIC POLICY, PRIVATE ADVOCACY: AN ASIAN EXAMPLE

A policy perspective on health system reform relevant to communities of color requires universal access regardless of residency, employment, citizenship status, or pre-existing conditions. All sectors of communities of color, including labor, consumers, community-based organizations, administrators, academics, psychologists, and human service workers, need to join in coalitions to impart this message to payers, legislators, and policymakers.

Within the Asian community in Boston, a specific strategy was used to inform and include the community in planning for changes under health care reform. South Cove Community Health Center collaborated with Region I, Office of Minority Health of the U.S. Public Health Service in sponsoring a Community Focus Group Forum on Health Care Reform in June 1994 (South Cove Community Health Center [SCCHC], 1994). The collaboration with public, private, and community agencies and individuals had several purposes. First, it was important to educate and inform the Asian community in the region about the rapid changes underway under health care reform.

Second, feedback from the Asian community was considered key to ensure that their needs would be addressed within any new health care delivery system. Lastly, the collection of data to be provided to key policymakers was needed to ensure inclusion in the planning and development of any health care reform measure. The following four questions were posed to the participants in an attempt to frame issues from a consumer and community perspective:

- What do you need for the health and well-being of your family?
- What do you do when you are sick?
- What is currently working well in terms of getting health care?
- What needs to be improved?

Community input identified the following important issues and concerns: 1) many Asians knew little about the rapid changes occurring in the health care environment; 2) high emphasis on the preference and common use of traditional methods of healing, including acupuncture and herbal remedies, and the questioning of its lack of reimbursement by third party payers; 3) emphasis on the importance of community education, outreach, and services in their primary language through bilingual providers, and case management services; and 4) emphasis on the importance of language and culture in the delivery of health care services given that the majority of Asian Americans in the United States are currently immigrants or refugees.

The overriding issue is that cultural competence is essential to ensure access for the Asian American population. The importance of culture is true even for Asian Americans who speak English although there is a tendency for many to ignore these aspects in the utilization of health care given the historic failure of the U.S. health care system to integrate culture in the delivery of services. Consequently, ethnocultural individuals and communities of color tend not to expect cultural relevance, sensitivity, and competence as a critical element of medical care practices. This point was underscored by the California Pan-Ethnic Health Network (CPEHN) in its development of guiding principles for a multicultural approach to health care system reform (California Pan-Ethnic Health Network, 1992). The irony which speaks to the importance of advocacy is highlighted by the fact that while California has been in the forefront in developing culturally competent criteria for health care reform, it is also the first state to pass a bill denying benefits to immigrants and the first to eliminate affirmative action in its university system.

PREVENTION AS A FOCUS

Inherent in a holistic approach and an emphasis on comprehensive service delivery is a focus on prevention. Prevention of illness, early identification, health education, community outreach, advocacy, health promotion, and early intervention are all important to a focus on prevention. Health promotion and disease prevention efforts should target stress-related disorders; alcohol, tobacco, and other drug abuse; injury control; lead poisoning; AIDS/HIV; chronic disease; immunizations; and violence and conflict resolution. Ethnic, racial, and gender health disparities should be taken into account in these areas for communities of color. Strategies for effective prevention can mean coalitions which go beyond local and/or geographic boundaries given that networks among communities of color often transcend traditional geographic boundaries.

An overriding principle of cultural competency is the support for ethnic-specific services. Application of this principle to prevention efforts would suggest the importance of initiatives which prevent delayed entry into care. For communities of color, appropriate linguistic support, bilingual providers, extended service hours, transportation, on-site child care, and "one stop shopping" in neighborhood family-oriented centers are among the characteristics promoting access and early entry to care (Herrell, 1994). As mainstream systems of care begin to co-opt the emphasis on multiculturalism and diversity historically advocated among communities of color, there is a growing insensitivity to the need for separateness of ethnic-specific services to address specific needs. The challenge is how to do this without creating a separate but inferior system, a racist and discriminatory system, or a disempowering system. It would appear that the current inequitable distribution of power in U.S. society for communities of color mitigates against separate systems being equal. The creation of new mega-systems in health care delivery can dilute the specific needs of communities of color.

A community driven and planned strategy of collaborative work among community-based organizations enhances the capacity of communities of color to build their infrastructure. Building from the ground up is an effective strategy to ensure that specific ethnoracial subgroup needs are met, community-based organizations survive, and larger, more established agencies remain relevant.

Commitment to consumer informed approaches, equitable distributions of power, institutional change, health advocacy and progressive policy, solidarity among diverse national, cultural, and local groups, and social and economic justice are necessary ingredients in this call for healthy praxis with communities of color (National Boricua Health Organization, 1990). A focus on prevention integrates these various principles and guidelines as suggestive of the holistic approach relevant to communities of color, the competency needed to serve them, and the comprehensiveness important to address their multiple and specific needs. To enhance the reader's awareness about such praxis, what follows is a specific example of a chemical dependency prevention approach for the Latino/a community. Again, it is intended to preserve the uniqueness important to a specific ethnic community while recognizing its relevance for other disenfranchised groups.

ATOD PREVENTION: A LATINO/A EXAMPLE

This example proposes empowerment-oriented health research as a means for developing community-based alcohol, tobacco, and other drug (ATOD) related disease prevention and health promotion programs for a Latino/a community. This approach identifies socioeconomic, cultural, and policy issues influencing ATOD use and abuse in a Latino/a population while recognizing intracultural diversity. Acknowledging current deficits in research infrastructure, it uses empowerment-oriented research and evaluation methods, and considers the politics of developing a health research agenda.

Since many Latino/a community-based organizations have had negative experiences with evaluators and researchers who contribute little to benefit the communities they study, particular emphasis is placed on participatory evaluation methods and research instruments intended to result in community empowerment. This empowerment agenda approach is modeled after Paulo Freire's work, which used an "empowerment" pedagogy that valued diversity and inclusiveness, highly experiential and interactive dialogue, and peer group discussion to emphasize social class and political considerations and achieve cultural competence. Freire's main philosophical theme was to give disenfranchised people the means and power to make decisions affecting their own lives and thus to empower communities.

An empowerment perspective for health promotion and disease prevention suggests that sociocultural competence is needed at all levels of research, including data collection, analysis, interpretation, reporting, and evaluation. The perspective is an explicitly political one, calling for systems change at all policymaking levels—individual, family, community, state, and federal—to promote self-determination. It posits that the very communities studied need to develop the skills to design, implement, evaluate, and control their own ATOD interventions utilizing a paradigm that recognizes family, community, and cultural strengths rather than just identifying deficits.

This approach is consistent with a community health psychology definition of prevention which would be sensitized to economic and cultural factors as potential agents of social change. Data collection would emphasize family values and common cultural beliefs important to Latinos/as in designing culturally competent and language appropriate disease prevention and health promotion programming for Latinos/as against ATOD abuse.

Intracultural Diversity

ATOD misuse and abuse, and its related problems of vehicular homicide, violence, cancer, HIV/AIDS, and other sexually transmitted diseases have recently been targeted for Latino/a community mobilization efforts. The interrelatedness of these multiple issues suggests that health promotion efforts become a catalyst for ATOD prevention by empowering people to address related community health concerns which disproportionately affect Latinos/as (e.g., crime reduction, rape, child and spouse abuse, teen pregnancy, injury prevention). Although prevention methods and programs have been developed to empower communities, still lacking are appropriate and competent community evaluation techniques and instrumentation to measure their process, outcome, and impact. This is particularly true for Latinos/as, who suffer twice over when prevention research is not made a priority and intracultural diversity is not recognized appropriately in the design of assessment tools and evaluation instruments (De La Cancela, 1995b).

Critical issues and meaningful inquiry to foster a specific and relevant understanding of Latino/a health-related concerns will be emphasized over providing comprehensive descriptions. Emphasis will also be on those issues systematically ignored by researchers and evaluators working with Latino/a communities in the past. Although Latino/a subgroups are proud of their cultural identity and heritage, not all actively amass knowledge of their social realities. In order to evaluate how a particular intervention has empowered a Latino/a community, a baseline measure is needed of how knowledgeable community members were about local, regional, and national leaders or organizations working on their behalf. Assessment of a specific Latino/a community's attitudes toward other Latino/a groups or towards the specific concerns of Latino/a men, women, youth, the aged, parents, families, migrants, immigrants, and undocumented or homeless transients is also required to determine if a Latino/a community-building health promotion has enhanced subgroup sensitivity to special populations within their own or other subgroups.

Although 67% of Latinos/as in the United States are U.S. born, differences in primary language spoken, and dialects among them significantly impact disease prevention, evaluation, and instrumentation strategies. Regional differences, idiomatic speech, slang, and monolingual or bilingual skills must be assessed to determine the utility and meaningfulness of audiovisual health promotion materials such as training films, instructional videos, slides, or audio cassette tapes. Linguistic differences also influence levels of assertiveness and the degree to which Latinos/as appear empowered in an individual interview or evaluation focus group (De La Cancela, 1995b).

Prevention research is often confounded by two variables. Racial heterogeneity among Latinos/as leads to some being misclassified in data collection as members of other ethnic-racial groups. The generally depressed socioeconomic standing of Latinos/as leads to confusion of social class with racial, ethnic, or gender issues in the analysis and interpretation of data. The U.S. Census Bureau's definition of Hispanics, for example, includes people coming from more than 20 countries; yet, the diversity of Latinos/as is not acknowledged by federal agencies since public health data for specific Latino/a subgroups is almost nonexistent. Illustrative is the lack of specific data on ATOD utilization and morbidity among Central and South Americans or Dominicans. Similarly, only 25 of the 300 *Healthy People 2000* objectives contain Latino/a-specific components; among the objectives lacking a Latino/a focus are tobacco use and substance abuse (Delgado & Estrada, 1992).

Recognition of Latino/a diversity suggests that effective disease prevention, intervention, and control programs would develop materials in Spanish and English or bilingual combinations that respond to the linguistic skill or preferences of the target subgroups—Yaqui or Mayan Indian dialects, Spanglish or calo of Latino/a urban youth. Efforts would be made to reach a mobile family-centric population and those Latinos/as who identify as people of color, as well as those who do not (De La Cancela, 1995b).

Research Paradigms: Infrastructure deficits

Adverse effects on evaluation of disease prevention and health promotion programs for Latinos/as result from shortages of Latinos/as in major health policy, management, and administration positions, and as prevention researchers. Consequently, most research involv ing Latinos/as has been conducted by non-Latinos/as, who are often insensitive to sociocultural nuances in their data collection. Their findings tend to reinforce negative stereotypes, perpetuate myths about Latino/a health and health care use, and provide misinformation. This is especially true when they ignore cultural coping skills or positive health practices that may be helpful in improving the status of all U.S. residents (National Hispanic Health Policy Summit, 1992).

One research infrastructure weakness is the inadequacy of dissemination of results. When culturally appropriate disease prevention research has occurred, findings are often published in journals, government documents, or technical program reports to which the Latino/a family and community, many policymakers, and front line workers have little access (De La Cancela, 1995b).

Specific Latino/a concerns also exist regarding the culturally appropriate nature of instrumentation used in the evaluation of disease prevention and health promotion interventions. Many of the commonly used instruments have an individual focus, implying that different behavior is primarily the fault of the individual (e.g., self-esteem scales). As such, they do not allow prevention evaluators to determine the role of racism, sexism, or sociopolitical and economic oppression on the Latino/a person or community (Grace, 1992). English language questionnaires and surveys used to collect information on Latino/a populations are also often loosely translated, lack standardization, and have poor statistical validation with Latino/a populations and subpopulations (De La Cancela, 1995b).

Additionally, evaluators sometimes merge or combine data collected using both Spanish and English surveys without pilot testing or statistically validating the content equivalency of both surveys (Casas, 1992). Finally, prevention research often does not pay adequate attention to sociocultural and group-specific attitudes, perceptions, expectation, or values (Marin, Amaro, Eisenberg & Opava-Stitzer, 1992) so that multiple data sources, including key Latino/a community informants are not tapped, e.g., clergy, spiritualists, "santeros," *bodega* owners, and other informal leaders (Casas, 1992; Marin et al., 1992).

These research infrastructure problems can be remedied by increasing the number of Latino/a prevention researchers in the ATOD area. U.S. Department of Health and Human Services or the U.S. Public Health Service, for example, might develop specific support programs for pre/post-doctoral training of Latino/a preventive services evaluators, as well as increasing Latino/a participation in all aspects of the research grants funding process. State educational, institutional, and professional associations and other governmental

ATOD concerned health agencies can develop courses, seminars, continuing education offerings and conferences on prevention evaluation methods for Latino/a populations (Marin, et al., 1992). Efforts to increase the number of Latino/a and non-Latino/a individuals who are skilled both in the areas of program evaluation and cultural competence must also be expanded (Orlandi, 1992).

More appropriate strategies for dissemination of research reports and communication of health information would include distribution of summary fact sheets and press releases in a timely manner to Latino/a community based organizations (CBOs), local, and national Latino/a organizations and legislators. The use of audiovisual materials such as VHS videos are especially recommended for providing information to CBOs. It may also be culturally appropriate to share prevention service delivery outcomes and results in family and community forums (Grace, 1992).

The Politics of Evaluation

Recent research findings suggest that effective prevention intervention targeted to Latino/a populations requires the establishment of a means for the community to generate the focus of the intervention (Munoz, 1982). Indeed, the community organization (CO) approach recognizes that there is not one Latino/a community but many different Latino/a subgroups. Each has varied social arrangements which require preventionists to earn the respect of community members while avoiding creating dependencies on the preventionists (McKeown, Rubenstein & Kelley, 1987). In recognizing that Latinos/as are not monolithic groups, the CO approach also acknowledges that Latinos/as have different sociopolitical views on various ATOD intervention issues such as methadone maintenance programs, drug-free treatment availability, switching to noninjection forms of drug use, and moderated drinking education programs.

Sociopolitical concerns impacting on Latino/a ATOD disease prevention include the likelihood that many Latinos/as listen more carefully to a health promotion message emanating from people of color than one coming from Caucasian, male, middle class authorities. Because governmental planning and public health policy have been historically rooted in institutionalized racism, ethnocentrism, heterosexism, and classism, some Latinos/as are distrustful of "new" attempts to eradicate ATOD among Latinos/as. More specifically, these suspicions often arise from the researcher's inability to provide follow-up treatment once people have been screened, insensitivity to psychocultural aspects of *verguenza* (shame) connected with

ATOD use, and Latinos/as' historical lack of access to treatment services due to sexism, classism, racism, or linguistic barriers. Therefore, it is important for prevention researchers to acknowledge the existence of "nonpathological" conspiracy theories, genocidal fears, and distrust regarding ATOD interventions within Latino/a communities (De La Cancela, 1989a).

Prevention practitioners should also remember that even though Latinos/as have been scapegoated and stereotyped for their ATOD use, they are inherently no less prejudicial than other cultural groups. Latino/a health promotion must be tailored to each subgroup's self-identification, as the community may discredit or avoid prevention efforts associated with another ethnic racial group.

Awareness of institutional racism can also lead preventionists to the realization that there is no such thing as a *neutral* disease prevention, health promotion, community intervention, or evaluation process. Evaluation research can either facilitate the integration of Latinos/as into the "logic" of the dominant system, i.e., conformity to the system; or it can contribute to critical consciousness through which people deal critically and creatively with their social reality, and discover how to participate in the transformation of their community (Sotomayer, 1985).

A political view of evaluation suggests that Latino/a researchers can unwittingly function as agents of social control, and therefore, they should examine the theoretical models from which their evaluation practices stem (Trader, 1977). Relevant questions include: Does the theory subtly perceive Latinos/as to be inferior? Can the theory permit shared control of the prevention evaluation process? Are historical, political, economic, and other societal factors seen as contributory to health behavior? Is the theory self-critical, nonstatic, and nondogmatic in its applications?

If the answers to these questions have negative consequences for Latinos/as, then researchers are not utilizing theoretical models that are culturally competent. In fact, they are using models that lead to intervention evaluations that are disempowering. Prevention interventions that subscribe to community empowerment will include community meetings to elicit community input, small group and family work to reinforce family values, and individual counseling that examines the effects of the "isms" on self-esteem and daily living. Interventions consisting of team-building exercises, family preservation, relational skills building, conflict resolution training, examining internalized oppression, and challenging Latino/a identity definitions, can also be utilized (De La Cancela & Sotomayer, 1993).

Empowerment-oriented Evaluation

The mutual participation of people in group action and dialogue enhances their control and ability to change their own lives. The empowerment-oriented evaluation identified above promotes Latino/a peoples' participation and control over their lives in their community and larger society. It promotes an examination of the effectiveness of disease prevention practices in targeting individual, family, group, and structural change. Empowerment-oriented evaluation looks beyond measurable goals and objectives; rather it examines whether a participatory process has taken place that engages people in critical evaluation of the causes of ATOD use as the basis for community action (De La Cancela, 1995b).

An application of these principles of empowerment-oriented evaluation to prevention is outlined in Appendices 2.1 and 2.2; examples of learning activities to engage participants and enhance their collective evaluation skills. They build on Freire's pedagogical method, as a process involving dialogue between equals in which groups of people reflect upon aspects of their reality, look behind these immediate problems to their root causes, examine the implications and consequences of these issues, and develop a plan of action to deal with them (Minkler & Cox, 1980). See Appendices 2.3 and 2.4 for examples of how participants might be stimulated to develop empowerment-oriented action plans.

Paulo Freire's ideas, adapted to prevention intervention, suggest that evaluators ask whether targeted individuals emerge as subjects and actors in their lives and society. Has the prevention program staff listened to the felt themes of the families in the community? Has there been participatory dialogue about the themes using a problem-posing method? Have actions taken place based upon the above? Empowerment-oriented evaluators recognize that prevention services modeled along Freire's approach will have multiple targets of change, be complex, require greater resources, and need longer time frames for reaching solutions.

Applied to ATOD disease prevention evaluation, an empowerment oriented approach suggests that preventionists take on the role of facilitators or "teacher-learners" who tune into the cultural values and "vocabular universe" of the target group through participant observation. They should work with small groups and families in search of "generative themes," i.e., key words reflective of a subgroup's hopes and concerns. They should then synthesize these themes, codify them in visual images, and give these symbols back to the group for decoding through "cultural circles." Within these cultural circles, the evaluator as facilitator or "coordinator-questioner," examines along with the group the causes, issues, implications, and possible solutions to the ATOD problems identified by the community. Suggested community health psychology interventions flowing from this method will promote the role of evaluators as a client to tune into the vocabular universe and become participant observers in the intervention program (Whalen, Tormala, & Osborne, 1976); it will prevent them from entering programs as ethnocentric cultural invaders who either overtly assess differences as deficits or covertly negate cultural diversity by claiming neutrality. These methods encourage the use of qualitative data in the cultural and political domain, when quantitative data is absent or inadequate, that can contribute to evaluation of sociopolitical prevention and intervention (De La Cancela, 1995b).

Two examples are the use of salsa music or Latino/a rappers to provide media messages in the cultural vocabulary of Latino/a youth, and the incorporation of prevention and family empowerment themes into murals created by Latino/a youth. These messages can decode the environmental racism of ATOD marketing and advertising which specifically targets Latinos/as in culturally oriented ways by depicting alcohol and tobacco use as normative family activities (De La Cancela, 1991b, 1991a). Musical and artistic vehicles can also utilize generative themes on the individual use of ATOD and tell the story of how the increasing number of Latinos/as suffering from cancer is related to the slick advertising of alcohol and tobacco products.

An ATOD-related area in which such biopsychosociocultural competent interventions have developed and which we can look to heuristically is AIDS treatment and prevention (De La Cancela & McDowell, 1992). Here we find individual, family, and community empowerment interventions that acknowledge the personhood, family, or community identification of target audiences by: encouraging participation in decision making (McKusick, April, 1991), advocating for increased protection of confidentiality (McKusick, May, 1991); teaching people how to make bureaucratic systems work for them (M. Smith, 1991); mobilizing audiences to negotiate health maintenance practices; and engaging in constructive confrontation in the service of health. Latinos/as can similarly benefit from proactive development of family support networks, mediation of their patient-provider communication, and control in disease prevention, health promotion, health service, and research.

Toward that end, the following questions and those presented in Appendix 2.5 can be utilized by evaluation researchers to assess the responsiveness of prevention intervention efforts to an empower-ment-oriented agenda:

1) Has a pre-intervention needs assessment been conducted that in-cluded Latino/a members diversified by their age, gender, race, sexual orientation, acculturation, nativity, citizenship, religion, marital status, family composition, extended kinship networks, social class, education, reading level, occupation, community ac-tivism, and ATOD use?
2) Have Latino/a community personnel been identified who facili-tate access to, use of, and effectiveness of the program?
3) Have specific Latino/a ATOD-related instruments been created in collaboration with Latino/a community members?
4) Have members of the target audiences been trained to conduct or participate meaningfully in disease prevention evaluation activi-ties?
5) Have interventions built in cultural, family, or community strengths to improve health promotion activities?
6) Has the intervention program provided or required any training to enhance the cultural competence of its administrators, profes-sional staff, board, or community members? (Kim, McLeod, & Shantzis, 1992)
7) Do participants feel empowered to establish community-based partnerships with local governmental and nonprofit agencies?
8) Have any long term meetings or agendas been put forward as a result of the intervention, or changes in community and family participation occurred, or plans for future community actions been developed?

CONCLUSION

In identifying strategies and mechanisms for meeting health care needs of communities of color, health systems reform is critical. In looking at an ideal health services program, certain principles stand out. These include: community-oriented services, community em-powerment, a holistic approach, and collaboration to ensure univer-sal access to a culturally competent system of care. Moreover, advocacy and prevention within a paradigm of empowerment ori-ented evaluation are essential to promote systems change given the historical "isms" which have posed barriers to accessing care. Pre-vention is at the core of these strategies and mechanisms given the interrelatedness of social, cultural, environmental, and public health problems and the importance of early intervention. However, it is important to recognize the intracultural diversity among communities of color lest we magnify those sociocultural attributes that may contribute to poor health, while ignoring concrete social, cultural, and economic realities (Rendon, 1984). Other consequences include culturally out-of-phase programs disastrously missing their targeted objectives, and wasted resources.

The importance of diversity extends to divergent political views on preventive services and evaluation within communities of color which include: views that disease prevention/health promotion efforts are yet another "Anglo" bureaucratic intrusion (Tafoya, 1991); conspiracy theories and fears that Caucasian health workers, trainees, and researchers may be "experimenting," are prejudiced against, or neglectful toward them (Kolata, 1991); and differing responses to disease prevention/health promotion messages (Salas Rojas, 1992).

While approaching change from the different perspectives of advocacy and prevention, many of the issues inherent in this chapter's Latino/a and Asian examples are shared by communities of color. Diversity within each of the communities of color is often not recognized; census labels are meaningless when skin color is not easily identified by others. For example, Asians are sometimes classified as Asian when they are born, but are classified as white, unknown, or other when they die since race is reported by mothers at birth, but by the undertaker at death. The inadequacy of data characterizing communities of color, the lack of ethnographic approaches to identify critical variables, and the poor understanding of family, community and cultural issues or protective factors among ethnic populations make for inadequate approaches to systems reform. This can lead to a failure to ensure competency in serving diverse populations or to allocate resources in the area of prevention.

Since public policy and successful advocacy is often influenced by research and data, it is important to train psychologists to conduct culturally competent research. They must be critical consumers of research and related social policy since conducting and disseminating research yields a significant amount of power (Harrell, 1995). As both examples demonstrate, racism must be treated as an important variable in evaluating the inadequacy of systems of care in being responsive to communities of color. Overemphasis on comparative approaches where ethnic populations are compared against Caucasians and the simplified reasoning of generalizing from statistical aggregates to individuals (Gary, 1978) result in negative and inappropriate characterization of communities of color. Considerations for culturally competent research include the importance of knowing historical and current sociopolitical contexts; using qualitative methodologies and designs; attending to trust and credibility issues; avoiding the use of negative stereotypes and pathologizing labels; recognizing the limitations of linear models; acknowledging biases in the interpretation of results; and giving back to the community (Harrell, 1995).

Complicating the development of strategies and mechanisms for meeting the health care needs of communities of color is the fact that research by psychologists of color is often published in nonpeer-reviewed journals because they allegedly do not meet the criteria of many peer-reviewed journals. While mainstream psychologists might argue that the quality is not good enough, those viewing from the perspective of communities of color might also argue that the criteria used in peer-reviewed journals are biased by perspectives irrelevant to communities of color. Such arguments are a challenge to the field and raise questions about the inadequacies of the current publication system and its failure to disseminate community-generated data, community health psychology perspectives, and information on ethnocultural and racial variables. Consequently, community-generated data and ethnocultural perspectives fail to become disseminated into the mainstream for promoting public policy or health systems change. The consequences of conducting culturally incompetent and thus potentially unethical research are considerable in reinforcing a system which fails to meet the needs of disenfranchised populations in U.S. society.

Community health psychology, with its emphasis on prevention, empowerment-oriented evaluation, and culturally competent policy and planning for a diverse population, has much to offer the fields of public health, human service, and mental health. Community health psychologists can consciously and intentionally combat the institutional racism evident in past theory, research, and practice by institutionalizing compassion toward people of color. Operationally, this means developing biopsychosocial and culturally competent interventions that are in sociopolitical collaboration with and inclusive of communities of color (De La Cancela, 1991b). It also means rejecting paternalistic service models, and promoting the recognition and transfer of competence in the individual, family, community, and cultural contexts of people of color to promote systems reform. The strategies, mechanisms, and philosophy for meeting the health care needs of communities of color must engage, mobilize, and empower those we serve (Szapocznik, 1994).

COMMENTARY

Pamela Jumper Thurman

*Quality health care is a critical issue for all. For minority popula-
tions, however, unique challenges are added. In the past, these challenges have not been met effectively, resulting in, as the authors
point out, decreased access to and acceptability of health care
among the poor and biopsychosocially underserved. It is with this
concept that this chapter begins to build toward a strong basis for a
closer examination of our changing health care system and the need
for holistic and comprehensive health services for minority populations. For the sake of the people we represent, it is imperative that
we remain current with new health initiatives and maintain a high
level of knowledge related to the health interests of the many diverse
ethnic groups. Then, as minority professionals, we must take this
one step further to become proactive in establishing and implementing quality and holistic systems of care that are attentive to the issues inherent in the many diverse ethnic groups.*

*This chapter clearly addresses the issues relevant to development
of the kinds of strategies that will impact national public policy
while giving concrete examples of programs that have a higher potential for success and impact on a community level as well. The authors are not afraid to take on the potentially controversial issues as
well—universal access to health care for undocumented residents,
for example.*

*Certainly this is a very timely publication. Many states are cur-
rently beginning the move toward restructuring the various state and
federally funded medical programs. It has been pointed out that
those who are able to access primary and comprehensive health
care increase their odds of preventing diseases or detecting them in
early states. However, historically, this accessibility and early detec-
tion has been a difficulty for minority people. They must overcome
various cultural barriers to access this type of care. The authors
point out that an ideal health care program for communities of color
would ensure universal access, comprehensive services, universal
coverage, and cultural competence. But what is significant about
this chapter is that they take these concepts even further by discussing how each component of the system can become actively involved in family, community, societal, and political arenas to
facilitate change.*

*American Indians are very likely the only ethnic group that have
had an entire system allocated to providing health care. Early efforts
left much to be desired. Care was fragmented and little effort was*

made to break down the cultural barriers. Today's hospitals and clinics are more sophisticated and most offer various facets of health care in one location, but, much still needs to be done in providing truly holistic health care. Some of the steps already taken include efforts to recruit American Indian staff and, in some areas, to utilize the services of traditional healers. In fact, this inclusion of healers is quite in line with the authors' discussion related to developing strategies that build connections with communities of color. They discuss two programs that have made successful connections by using a systems approach that involves various segments of the community, including even corporate business and the local chambers of commerce. They ground their case for a community-driven collaborative strategy firmly in the principles and guidelines that have created success in the programs presented in the chapter.

These guidelines also extend to the areas of culturally congruent program evaluation and the need for participatory methods and designs that empower communities. In fact, the chapter speaks to the nature of evaluation as a method by which communities of color can facilitate change and be a collaborative component in the measurement and use of the outcome data.

Finally, a very important element raised by the authors relates to the need for effective dissemination of information, whether program evaluation or research. It is significant to note that when effective models or research data have been developed, findings are published in journals, government documents, or technical program reports to which front line workers seldom have access. As a result, very powerful interventions with great potential for change may never reach the communities that need them.

Community-oriented services and cultural competence in health care are indeed critical. This chapter provides an integral component for the development of strategies to overcome the barriers in delivery of holistic and culturally congruent health services to communities of color. We have a great responsibility to lead others toward progress. Collaboratively, it can be done.

APPENDIX 2.1[1]

BUILDING SUPPORT
THROUGH COLLECTIVE ACTION

1) List your fears about ATOD use/misuse here.
2) What is the experience of ATOD users/abusers in this community, e.g., isolated, stigmatized?
3) Identify people you can turn to for ATOD prevention intervention help here.
4) List things you can offer others in exchange for their support.
5) How can families be strengthened or supported to deal more effectively with problem substance use behavior?

APPENDIX 2.2

EMPOWERMENT: UNDERSTANDING
THE SOURCES OF POWER(LESSNESS)

System	How Latino/a Communities are Empowered/Disempowered	Self-Esteem Impact
• Health • Schools • Housing Authority • Public Assistance • Peers • Family • Job/Employer		

---

1. Appendices 2.1 to 2.5 have been adapted from Richie, 1992.

APPENDIX 2.3

THE CAUSES OF ATOD MISUSE/ABUSE

1) List the reasons Latinos/as use ATOD.
2) Go back and be sure you included social and institutional factors as well as individual and familial ones. Now categorize the list.
3) What do institutions gain/lose from Latino/a ATOD use/misuse?

MY ACTION PLAN

Now develop an action plan for each category and write your plan below.

Individual/family changes I can make:
Social messages I can work for/against:
Institutional policies I can develop/confront:

APPENDIX 2.4

EMPOWERED ATOD PREVENTION
INTERVENTION ACTION PLANS

Systems I expect to work well/badly with	Method of (dis)empowerment	My plan

Potential positive(negative) consequences:

Anticipated benefits/losses:

APPENDIX 2.5

QUESTIONS FOR EVALUATING LATINO/A EMPOWERMENT-ORIENTED ATOD PREVENTION INTERVENTION PROGRAMS

1) Does the program address issues related to the disenfranchising or cultural oppression of Latinos/as?
2) Are ATOD issues presented in a manner that can be easily understood by large groups of people?
3) Do ATOD prevention-intervention efforts expose the injustice of discrimination?
4) Who is in opposition to this community program's prevention-intervention action?
5) What community agencies are in support of it?
6) What particular community action/series of actions are successful in achieving the Latino/a ATOD prevention-intervention objective?
7) Are these actions consistent with an empowering vision of the future?
8) What resources are needed to do what the program wants to do, and do participants have those resources? If not, how do they get them?

3

Psychosocial and Cultural Impact on Health Status

Victor De La Cancela,
Yvonne M. Jenkins, and Jean Lau Chin

GENERAL CONSIDERATIONS:
DIFFERENTIAL MANIFESTATIONS

Since almost every aspect of human behavior seems to be either modifiable or influenced by social, cultural, and psychological factors, clinicians should examine how health care orientations, utilization, and treatment may be affected. This chapter presents some "cultural idioms of distress" (Kleinman, 1980) and social uses of the sick role that health practitioners might possibly encounter in their treatment of disease and illness. Such information can be of use in clinical interventions and evaluations of therapy over a long period of time.

It should be remembered that Western health practitioners form their own "cultural" systems with a specialized language, symbolic rituals, and modes of constructing reality. As such, patient-practitioner interactions are moments when different cultural systems come into contact and therefore require compromises and negotiations. Whereas previous studies in this area have emphasized the psychological or cultural factors involved in these interactions, this chapter attempts where possible to reference social economic aspects.

It has been suggested that the source of disease and illness may be social rather than pathogenic, and practitioners may come to realize that certain"diseases" may be dealt with more effectively through social interventions. Indeed, the provision of adequate health care must involve both micro and macro analyses and approaches. Part of the necessary combinations involve the health practitioner learning to follow certain rules: conveying respect; listening carefully; explaining procedures carefully; showing active and authentic interest in the patient's cultural background; not patronizing patients; and understanding that fear of hospitals, values of endurance and self-healing, lack of money, and previous *care-less* treatment can combine to prolong suffering and prevent care (Kemnitzer, 1980). A large and probably more important component of the process is the delivery of health care from a philosophical orientation that states that comprehensive, unfragmented, individualized health care must be made accessible to all who seek it and is controlled by consumers themselves (Source Collective, 1974).

Historically, healers promote the physical and psychological well-being of individuals in most societies. This is true of contemporary U.S. health providers, yet their efforts are often challenged by the diverse presenting complaints encountered in a pluralistic society. Additionally, most providers are unfamiliar with the different health care orientations of various ethnic, racial, and social populations.

The intent of this chapter is to inform practitioners of health care orientations which impact the patient and practitioner's therapeutic relationship. These different explanatory models of etiology, anatomy, physiology, nutrition, psychology, and intervention at times lead to differential use of health care sectors. Additionally, health care practitioners are asked to free themselves of ethnocentrism and class biases as expressed in medico-centricity (Kleinman, Eisenberg, & Good, 1978). By educating ourselves we can avoid viewing persons or communities of diversity as problematic, difficult, or abnormal and increase acceptance, understanding, and culturally competent care. We can ally with the patient to effect changes based on a negotiated and empowerment approach to health care rather than one of conflict, rejection, and subjugation (De La Cancela, 1990a).

Community health psychology is our preferred approach for alliances with ethnocultural diversity in health status, since it offers an environmental and psychosocial analysis that moves from clinical psychology's concern with individual patient histories to more collectivist, community informed, and population-based perspectives of health care practices, codes, and rituals. Community health psychology provides a pathway to a public health psychology that frames the understanding of health and illness in interdisciplinary behavioral sciences, advances the practice of health maintenance and reaches a larger segment of the medically undeserved. Its importance includes the use of epidemiology to examine the demographic characteristics, diet, environment, and behavior of groups of people to discover possible causal links between these factors and disease development. Epidemiology's aim is to uncover statistically significant correlations between certain factors and disease. These factors then are labelled "risk" factors which are targeted for intervention. The varied factors examined by epidemiology are those that may influence the spread of infectious disease, predispose individuals to certain types of trauma, morbidity, or mortality, and/or place them at risk of psychosocial disruption. Psychocultural aspects of all these factors must be considered in order to determine comprehensively the multifactorial causes of certain disease and to plan interventions that attend to these causes (Marmot, 1981). The importance of epidemiology is its ability to examine demographic characteristics of groups and correlate them with health status. Psychosocial and cultural diversity in epidemiology is relevant to community health psychology in terms of the multiple needs that people have for case management, counseling, health education, social services, and advocacy to overcome the cross-cultural challenges and obstacles of the Western medical care system. It also contributes to efforts to sort out genetic from environmental factors by studying trends between immigration status and health status.

ANATOMY AND PHYSIOLOGY

Most people have different conceptualizations of the major organs in their bodies and what their functions are. For example, the stomach may be thought of as consisting of the whole or only part of the abdominal cavity, or the heart as encompassing all of the thoracic cavity. These patient attributions may interfere with providers' abilities to pinpoint the actual site of pain or to understand the patient's subjective sense of distress (Helman, 1985).

Additionally, clients have cultural views of anatomy and physiology that affect them, as illustrated by beliefs held by some Latina women who fear bathing or swimming during their menstrual period because the "cold" water might clot the "hot" blood, thereby interrupting the flow which might then cause a "back-up." Such fears may lead these women to avoid certain methods of contraception that cause changes in menstruation. Some Asians believe that you should not go to sleep with damp hair because the pores will reabsorb moisture and cause rheumatism. Some African American women have similar beliefs that associate exposure to dampness with tuberculosis.

Shared cultural views of "hot" and "cold" in some Asian and Latino cultures not only reflect psychosocial values, they also prescribe important rituals in the healing process and in maintaining health. For example, in Asian cultures, food and body states are defined in terms of their hot or cold properties. The importance of balance in the body fluids and its hot and cold properties are also considered critical to health and well being. This balance is achieved through nutrition and herbal tonics which help to restore balance. Specifically, physical and psychological health is believed to be influenced by yin and yang qualities, or "hot and cold." Deficiencies caused by the failure of one to regulate the other can be corrected by tonics and herbal soups, which have played significant roles in the healing practices of Chinese families. Herbal soups routinely used in cooking and often served as part of a meal have distinct yin qualities (water, female) to balance an overabundance of yang qualities (fire, male). Thus, many foods are identified by their "hot and cold" properties separate from their nutritional value, thereby dictating diet patterns among many Chinese families.

It is important to highlight that some cultural views of anatomy and physiology are more than superstitions to those who hold them. These are revered beliefs and prized knowledge passed from one generation to another, which provide important connections and have symbolic value even as they sometimes reflect alternative medical and health sophistication related to blocked access to health education and quality health care. Clinicians should avoid aiding the perpetuation of racism, sexism, classism, and discrimination by ridiculing or dismissing such information. Instead they should explore any beliefs consumers may have to determine how likely a patient is to follow prescribed practices. Additionally, we are only now beginning to find scientific proof for some of these practices and beliefs. It should also be remembered that the psychological value of faith and empowerment through holding of these beliefs contributes to their importance in holistic healing.

PERSPECTIVES OF DIFFERENT HEALTH CARE SECTORS

The accepted visible health care sectors of clinicians (e.g., clinics, hospitals, mental health centers) may not be the only possible ones, as viewed by the client. Different sectors of health care representing different accepted orientations to health care have been identified in the literature. Although some may view these sectors along a

continuum of increasing technical expertise and scientific sophistication, we need to recognize and examine the mythology and ritual
associated with all sectors. In doing so, we may find the similarities
greater than the differences between these different health care sectors. The significance of these sectors is that patients make their
health choices in a cultural context, and will seek out providers
with demonstrated expertise in cross-cultural health care (Walker,
1994). Thus, in an increasingly multicultural and health costs-
conscious society, all health practitioners must do more than recognize differences. They must learn to equip themselves with cultural
competence tools, including knowledge, skills, and abilities to
serve empowered consumers from diverse ethnoracial, national and
cultural groups (Walker, 1994). A brief review of different sectors
follow (De La Cancela, 1990a).

Popular

Ill-health is often first recognized and defined by relatives, friends,
neighbors, or workmates, who collectively comprise the popular
health care sector. One positive aspect of this sector is that access to
health care occurs within the immediate and extended family arena
between people linked by ties and where patient and healer mani-
fest complementary assumptions about health and illness (Chrisman, 1981). Another advantage is that therapeutic encounters occur
without fixed rules governing behavior or defined settings; indeed,
roles may even be reversed such that today's patient is tomorrow's
healer. Credentials are usually based on one's own experience with
specific illnesses rather than education or special occult powers.
However, this sector also can have negative effects on the patient's
health. For example, the family may exert pressure not to disclose
personal matters to "outsiders" (Rosado, 1980). Similarly, patients
may be advised against following suggested medical procedures
(Snow, 1978).

Additionally, use of poisonous substances may be self or family
prescribed, for example, mixing chlorine bleach with water, drinking mercury, and placing turpentine on sugar cubes (C.S. Scott,
1974), or treating diarrhea with folk remedies that result in lead poisoning (Carrad, 1983).

Folk

In this sector, certain individuals *specialize* in forms of healing
which are either sacred or secular, or a combination of the two. They

include: bonesetters, midwives, herbalists, spiritual healers, clair-voyants, and shamans. The approach is usually holistic, and in-cludes inquiry about the patient's behavior, conflicts with other people and physical symptoms. Folk practitioners provide explana-tions and treatment for feelings of guilt, shame, or anger, by pre-scribing prayer and repentance (Helman, 1985).

Compared to Western practitioners folk healers with their familiar rituals are viewed by clients as providing: more time with patients; warmth and authentic connection; informality; use of everyday lan-guage; rapid accessibility to services; the involvement of family and community members in familiar settings; the placing of responsibil-ity for illness beyond individual control; and similar social class, economic positions, and cultural background. Also, their services often are provided at little or no cost. Folk medicine skills are usu-ally acquired via apprenticeship, experience, spirit possession, being born within a "healing" family, and/or revelation (Snow, 1978). Healers abound in many societies as illustrated by the exis-tence of Latino/a *espiritistas*, *santeros*(as), and *curanderos(as)*; Na-tive American medicine men and shamans; Asian herbalists; Buddhist monks and acupuncturists; mediums and fortune tellers; root doctors, astrologers; polarity therapists; naturopaths; and faith healers (De La Cancela, 1978).

Allegedly, language barriers, transportation problems, and lack of cultural fit make these "providers" more palatable to some con-sumers than professional health providers. This may be true even when the professional providers themselves are bilingual-bicultural, for here possible sociopolitical antagonisms might exist—for exam-ple, an anti-Castro Cuban provider and a progressive Puerto Rican client (C.S. Scott, 1974). Additionally, many low-income ethnics see little profit in giving up folk remedies which have been supportive and accessible for generations in order to subscribe to the beliefs and practices of professional health systems to which they have little ac-cess (C.S. Scott, 1974). Finally, folk practitioners may be judged as more adept at treating certain folk illness such as fright (*susto*), weakness (*fatiga*), and nerves (*nervios*) than professional health providers since they do not stigmatize the patient in her help seek-ing (Rosado, 1980). For these reasons folk healers are often used si-multaneously with Western medicines. A negative aspect to this sector is that some folk healers use their reputations to extract money from the poor and gullible, and their alleged occult powers may be nearly as frightening to patients as illness itself (Snow, 1978).

Professional

Professional practitioners have organizations that maintain control over their fields of expertise, promote their interests, monopolize their knowledge, set criteria for admission into the field, and protect them from competition for consumers and reimbursements. The professional's main institutional structure is the hospital, where the patient is removed from friends, family, and community and converted into a "case." The hospital emphasis is on disease. Despite some recognition of a role for social service departments and mental health workers, there is often little, if any, reference to the home environment, religion, spirituality, or social status. Patients are often subjected to loss of control over their bodies, personal space, privacy, behavior, diet, use of time, and full knowledge of their condition. The relationships in hospitals are characterized by distance, formality, depersonalization, jargon, and brief conversations. Hospitals are often viewed by lay persons as a place where patients have no voice and die, and institutions with "foreign" codes and ritual.

Though hospital practitioners often are unaware of their rituals, such rituals permit practitioners to act autonomously and enable them to function in circumstances of ambiguity (Helman, 1985). These codes include:

1) entrance to certain areas being restricted to those properly costumed or considered to be of high status, importance
2) uniforms being worn to identify general roles in the hospital;
3) objects, space and people being classified as sterile or nonsterile, clean, dirty, or contaminated;
4) technical jargon;
5) privacy and confidentiality concerns;
6) dispassionate emotional reactions to medical conditions and parts of the human body; and
7) perfunctory interactions with relatives and friends of patients, which are permitted differential access to providers and the patient according to institutional classifications of kinship.

Within this setting the patient who expresses his concern and fears is often regarded as a hindrance to the smooth functioning of the hospital. Here the white coat symbolizes power to take a medical history, obtain intimate details of patients' lives, examine bodies, order tests, and prescribe medication or treatment. Beepers, prescription pads, stethoscopes, and name tags suggest healing power in the same way that religious artifacts do with popular and folk healers (Posner, 1986).

The exception to the traditional biomedical-oriented health care practitioner is probably the general, family, or primary care practitioner who may be a familiar figure in the community, takes part in local activities, uses everyday language, does check-ups, gives immunization and contraceptive advice, deals with marital and school problems, counsels, does home visits, and deals with more than one generation of a family. In essence this practitioner adheres to the hallmark of all healers—accessibility to all in need (Racer, 1980). This accessibility provides and maintains authentic connection and needs to be fashioned into a tool for use in culturally competent treatment, thereby becoming the key to care for people in the manner they are most likely to accept treatment.

Comparative psychocultural examination of the professional sector and community sector (popular and folk) suggests that access is either promoted or decreased by the codes and rituals present in both sectors and how these are viewed by the consumer. The challenge to health systems planners and managers is how to change their service delivery to be more accessible to the culturally different through incorporation of the best practices of the community sector.

CULTURAL DEFINITION OF COMMON DISORDERS

Health practitioners are often confronted with cases where psychological factors account for the illness. Indeed, it has been estimated that anywhere from 20 to 80%, averaging 50% of the typical health practitioner's caseload is made up of functional disorders for which no organic basis for illness exists. Surprisingly, the contemporary training of most health care practitioners leaves them ill-prepared for this reality. Hence, the following discussion of common presenting disorders is provided, with emphasis placed on the psychosocial and cultural influences, and suggested methods to gather information regarding these factors (De La Cancela, 1990b).

Asthma

Poor living conditions and the problems associated with poverty including crowding, poor ventilation, air pollution, poor heat, inadequate nutrition, and high infestations of insects (allergenic cockroaches and house dust mites) and parasites may be responsible for high rates of asthma among low-income clients (Sifontes & Mayol,

1976). Dusts, chemicals, and microbes can alter lung function by stimulating the immune system; houses that are deteriorating badly will have a higher count of insects and will also have excess dampness; poor people have little access to air conditioning that filters pollution; lack of heat and adequate nutrition contribute to frequent lung infections; and leaky and drafty doors and windows contribute to upper respiratory infections (Guarnaccia, 1981). Along with these stimulants from the physical environment, psychosocial stressors may add to the asthmatic's problems. These may include: family stress, high unemployment rates, serious housing problems, and discrimination (Guarnaccia, 1981). Additionally, tobacco dependence in the form of cigarette smoking and secondhand smoke adversely affect the asthmatic children of smokers. And the lack of access to preventive health care and routine primary care among low-income and poor populations has led to asthma, a condition that can be treated and controlled on an ambulatory care basis, being an alarmingly frequent presentation among Puerto Ricans and African Americans in hospital emergency rooms. For example, three times as many African Americans die of asthma than Caucasians (Villarosa, 1994).

From an individual perspective, patient management may be enhanced if the practitioner promotes patient education and self-care. For example, they can suggest use of nonallergenic bedding and involve the patient's family when possible in treatment efforts (Knapp, 1977). However, a more promising approach is for practitioners to engage in macro-level advocacy and social action that focuses attention on the social problems that give rise to this disease (De La Cancela, 1990b).

Substance Use Disorders

The ingestion of any chemical may have a symbolic aspect for those who take it (Helman, 1985). It may symbolize, for example, that the patient is ill, weak, or inadequate; that personal failures are due to illness; that the patient deserves sympathy and attention from family and friends; or that health practitioners are interested in the patient. Substance use may also symbolize hope for healing or cures. Drug use may be engaged in to improve social relationships, to relieve emotional distress or improve one's emotional state, or to rebel against or conform to social pressures. For some intoxication may be associated with virility, fashion, humor, escape, a sense of camaraderie or relational connection to others, or adulthood (O'Connor, 1975). Smoking has also been perceived as an indicator of maturity and as a stress reducer (Helman, 1985). Tobacco, peyote, marijuana, and other substance use are also part of the religious practices of some North and South American Indian and Rastafarian groups. Other cultural specific substance abuse includes beetle nuts among Pacific Islanders, chewing of coca leaves by indigenous peoples of South America, and the historical use of opium in China and among early Chinese Americans (Zane, Takeuchi, & Young, 1994).

From a therapeutic perspective, this suggests that discussions be held with users to determine *why* they engage in substance use behavior and thereby plan interventions that fulfill these needs in nondestructive ways (De La Cancela, 1990b).

Chronic Pain

Not all social or cultural groups respond to pain in the same way, for how people perceive pain, both in themselves and in others, and whether they communicate their pain to health practitioners, is often dependent on sociocultural factors like age, race, ethnicity, gender, sexual orientation, and social class (Webb, 1993). It is possible to exhibit pain behavior in the absence of a painful stimulus (hypochondriacs and malingerers) and not to exhibit such behavior in the presence of a painful stimulus (Fabrega & Tyma, 1976). This occurs because pain is essentially a private affair (Szasz, 1957), where observers are dependent on verbal and/or nonverbal signals from the person that she is in pain. Revealing that one is in pain also has to do with issues of pride and cultural conditioning.

Such communication is dependent on whether the person originates from a society where restraint, stoicism, and fortitude are valued, hence reserve is exhibited in the face of suffering; whether one's position in society has historically permitted helpseeking rather than self-caretaking; whether the pain is viewed as normal or abnormal; or whether it is viewed as divine punishment which must be experienced without complaint to expiate guilt (Helman, 1985). Additionally, the availability of potential healers also determines whether pain behavior will be displayed and in what setting, for individuals may respond sympathetically or punitively according to their roles vis-a-vis the sufferer (friend versus employer).

The developmental components of pain include (Engel, 1959): its function in infancy, where it leads to crying and may generate a comforting response from loving caretakers; in childhood, where pain and punishment are linked to being "bad" and pain may be associated with the expiation of guilt; and in later years, where pain may be associated with power, oppression, vulnerability, loss, and sexual experience. Practitioners should request a description of the pain, the circumstances under which it occurs, and the specific part of the body affected to determine its metaphorical meaning to the patient. In this way, patients' behavior can be analyzed to see if it is meant to ameliorate or intensify pain. Descriptions like "I just can't describe it," or dramatic elaborate imagery like "being jabbed," "burning," "bruised and torn," "eaten up," "electrical shocks," and other sensations described as boring, gnawing, pulling, biting, penetrating, crawling, and twisting are particularly meaningful in revealing the psychic processes at work in the pain experience (Engel, 1959).

Pain may also paradoxically occur when a positive life event has occurred or is imminent, as if the patient believes a price must be paid for happiness. Or it may occur to elicit a response from cold and distant or hostile family members who display affectionate responses only when the patient is ill. Some pain might have a history dating back to adolescent sexual conflicts, where it reflected guilt about sexual impulses and prevented or accompanied sexual activity. Pain may also accompany the mourning of loved persons or appear on the anniversaries of such losses, especially if the "lost" person was ambivalently or aggressively regarded. It may also appear in relation to threatened losses, such as the illness or departure of family members or friends, as a vehicle for re-establishing relationships. In some cases people have social networks that require admitting to psychic "pain" in order to continue membership, e.g., 12-step groups like Sexual Compulsives Anonymous, Co-Dependents Anonymous, and Incest Survivors Anonymous (Helman, 1985).

Finally, pain may be a product of somatization, a symptom of depression, hypochondriasis, or a result of operant conditioning where pain behaviors have been reinforced by the patient's environment and interaction with others (Fordyce, 1976). Pain may also be accidently associated with a harmless stimulus (classical conditioning) and continued by means of instrumental conditioning.

These considerations lead to recommendations that the complexity of pain be recognized and that treatment models include: positive reinforcement of more physical activity and fewer complaints on the part of patients; gaining the patient's cooperation and confidence toward rehabilitation; patient education about the nature of pain; biofeedback and relaxation exercises to encourage pain control; use of videotapes of ethnoracial and gender diverse patients coping with pain to encourage patient modeling; and group, family, and couples therapies to explore how pain is utilized as a vehicle of communication with others (Webb, 1983). We have found the utilization of poetry, folk songs, ethnic music, and art to be an important adjunct to the treatment of pain and stress among Latino/a and

African American clients. Sometimes framing an intervention or directive regarding stress or pain in the form of a metaphor, idiomatic expression, or cultural proverb is useful because it is respected, and commonly used to communicate scholarly thoughts or folk wisdom. An example is the use of a couplet (a two-phrase saying made up of four words each) with Chinese clients familiar with Confucian sayings. These artistic expressions serve as linguistic and nonverbal cultural triggers to memories of loss, catharsis, relaxation, and soothing feelings. An important referral resource in the case of pain is the cognitively and/or behaviorally trained bilingual-bicultural psychologist who can treat pain by manipulating stimuli after a thorough culture-informed behavioral analysis (De La Cancela, 1990b).

Hypertension

Known as the "silent killer," hypertension (high blood pressure) may impair or destroy vital organs—heart, brain, kidneys. Hypertension is often a contributory factor to heart attack, stroke, or other serious conditions that include kidney damage, diabetes, blindness or impaired vision. Particularly prevalent among African Americans, this disorder appears to have sociohistorical connections to the "middle passage," the deadly voyage that brought captured West Africans over the Atlantic to the Americas. Many died of dehydration and salt depletion secondary to diarrhea. Of those who survived, many retained salt, which is known to retain water and combat dehydration. It is thought that "the ability to retain salt may have passed from generation to generation" and made African Americans more "salt sensitive" so that blood pressure within this group is more likely to be influenced by salt intake (Villarosa, 1994).

Among other factors that contribute to the incidence of hypertension are: poverty, stress, obesity, unhealthy nutritional practices, excessive smoking, lack of preventive health care, inaccessibility to health education and healthy nutrition information. Poverty often limits access to quality health care. In addition, it limits access to some nutritious foods while making others high in salt and fat content readily available to the poor. For African Americans this, too, has origins in slavery when slave owners made the least desirable cuts of meat, often high in fat content, and low-cost filling foods available to slaves (Bass, Wyatt, & Powell, 1987). Some foods were extensively seasoned with salt and fried in saturated fat. Popular "soul food" cuisine continues to include some of these foods and methods of preparation and preservation, which are not limited to low-income communities where health education and nutrition information are often lacking. Perhaps the endurance of these patterns across socioeconomic classes is indicative of what has become their significance to African American tradition.

Psychological distress linked to daily exposure to societal disorders—racism, sexism, classism, prejudice, and discrimination, is commonly manifested by anger, anxiety, and depression. This exposure begins quite early in life and dictates African American socialization significantly. For some, survival is dependent on the ability to become estranged from disturbing emotions. Hypertension is often associated with internalization of such emotional states. Furthermore, obesity linked to stress-related eating and smoking, unhealthy food preparation, and diet deficiencies are linked to hypertension.

Vulnerability to hypertension is increased by inaccessibility to preventive health care, health education, and nutrition counseling. Without these services vital screening, self-monitoring, treatment, and adherence to health maintenance practices are unlikely.

In view of the critical impact of hypertension on the health of African Americans, it appears that the empowerment of this population to deal with the disorder must involve the following individual and community interventions: 1) accessible preventive health care, e.g., community-based and mobile units offering early screening at no cost to the homebound elderly, including blood pressure checks, diagnostic testing for heart disease, signs of mild stroke, kidney damage, and other related conditions; 2) health fairs and health education workshops offered in conjunction with African American churches, Afrocentric civic and service groups, community schools, and health centers; 3) nutrition counseling and education concerning the sociohistorical context of available food and methods of preparation to provide insight into how some choices and methods reflect the disenfranchisement of African Americans since slavery; 4) medically supervised weight loss intervention; 5) smoking cessation programs; and 6) socioculturally competent relaxation and stress reduction intervention.

At a macro level large-scale media campaigns are needed that educate communities of color about prevention of high risk factors associated with hypertension. Moreover, advocacy and social action focused on eradicating poverty and other social problems must become a priority for practitioners, health and mental health administrators, and legislators. Without this attention, such conditions will continue to impose barriers to timely and quality health care, and to contribute to the stress that increases vulnerability to developing hypertension.

Stress

The range of possible stressors experienced by patients is wide and includes: 1) discrimination related to language difficulties, racism, classism, sexism, and cultural shock/migration; 2) losses related to severe illness or trauma, wartime experiences, natural disasters, immigration, separation from family, divorce and marital conflict, and death; 3) occupational factors including promotions, un- and under-employment, retirement, job relocation, time pressure, interpersonal tension at work, financial difficulties, and changes in occupation; 4) loneliness and absence of meaningful connections to family or friends. Stress related to any of these events or conditions can be either causal or contributory to disease development, and can similarly influence illness in as much as it impinges on the patient's life space and social relationships (Helman, 1985). Social support and a sense of group cohesion appear to protect against stress as do certain cultural processes. For example, Latino/a family cohesion may enable the individual to better cope with the struggle of daily life (la lucha); the extended family network among African Americans may minimize stress through its support; and meditative and contemplative cultural values among Asians may be less conducive to stress than the White Anglo Saxon of ambitiousness, competitiveness, and concerns about material achievement (Helman, 1985).

Sociocultural beliefs, values, and practices can both increase the number of stressors an individual is exposed to, as well as the individual's response to them. These include a possibly different definition of what is a failure, loss of face, sense of shame, and bad behavior. For example, failure to "keep up with the Joneses" among Western consumers may result in subjective distress, while failure to "properly" marry off one's daughter may result in a sense of shame and loss of honor among some Latinos/as and Italians (Helman, 1985). Shame has particularly strong connotations across cultures. In Western cultures, it is usually experienced as an individual stressor. In Asian cultures, it is shared; the inclusion of family and others in one's shame is a phenomenon that magnifies the experience and psychological consequences of feeling ashamed. Thus, suicide has been a common solution for an individual to rectify and restore dignity to the family. Belief in hexes or curses can lead to "voodoo death" among the South Africans, Haitians, and Australians (Landy, 1977), and the unequal distribution of money in society is usually stressful to its poorer members. Other examples include: long-term admission to psychiatric settings or geriatric wards in Western settings, which can create a new set of stressors for patients at the same time that family members and friends withdraw from them, exclude them from their functions and activities, and regard them as objects of fear, shame, or irrevocable illness (Helman, 1985). A less extreme example of culturogenic stress is the damaging effect on health and behavior of certain diagnostic labels. For example, telling the patient: "You've got cancer," may lead the patient to assume behavior his reference group deems appropriate to sufferers of this condition. As such the labels lead to self-fulfilling prophecies (Waxler, 1977) since they provoke anxiety and foreboding.

Questions to use for exploring stress and the availability of social supports to the patient include: To whom can you talk when you need help? What would it take to make you feel okay? Additionally, sharing personal experiences with socially related tensions and stress can be helpful (De La Cancela, 1990b).

CULTURAL DIAGNOSIS OF MENTAL HEALTH ISSUES

A biopsychosocial perspective suggests that the majority cultural views of "normal" and "abnormal" when applied to ethnically diverse patients' beliefs, emotional states, or behaviors might ignore a universe of phenomena that are important in the patient's life and functioning. Given phenomena that at times include experiences of oppression, sexism, limited social roles, stereotypes, and lowered self and social esteem, it can be argued that diagnostic labelling can be a medicalized form of social control (Chin, De La Cancela, & Jenkins, 1993; Littlewood & Lipsedge, 1982).

Toward avoiding ethnocentric and class-bound labelling of patients, practitioners should briefly examine how intimately related are the patterns of social relations outside health care to the patient's condition. It appears that a society's economic and political issues are expressed in the patient's psychological state.

Nerves

Many low socioeconomic and ethnic clients often present to practitioners with the chief complaint of "nerves." This condition appears to include anxiety and varied somatic complaints (fainting, memory difficulties, weakness, or inability to work). For those who invoke this complaint, it carries a biological rather than emotional connotation and such patients view themselves in need of physical rather than psychiatric care. Many people claim to be born with "nerves" while others develop it in later life. They usually refer to their disorder by stating "I've got bad nerves." Whether nerves is a folk illness or a culture-bound syndrome is unclear, as is its relationship to anxiety or other psychiatric symptomology.

Six major features of "nerves" have been identified (Ludwig, 1982). They are:

1) *sense of inadequacy and nonassertiveness*—patients feel unsure about their judgements, do not speak out when offended, avoid conflicts with others;
2) *hapless*—patients fret and worry constantly about the most trivial things, yet feel that is the way of life;
3) *absence of social protest*—patients show amazingly little bitterness or resentment toward society. They do not complain about exploitation or repression and avoid antisocial, acting-out behavior. Some patients are unaware that they are exploited, oppressed, or marginalized;
4) *easy startle response* - patients frighten easily and are timid, high-strung, and jumpy. Sudden movements and loud noises alarm them;
5) *somatic nonspecificity*; and
6) *constricted world view*—life is monotonous and routine with an avoidance of novelty, strangers, or expanding of the social network. They have no close friends, and their knowledge about current or local events is vague. They have trouble maintaining sustained attention.

Some claim that among other diagnoses nerves represents: chronic anxiety without panic; mild depression without despair; a smattering of hypochondriasis; and an abundance of illness behavior (Ludwig, 1982). Prevention geared toward the young and future generations is often suggested as practitioners feel adults are too chronic to change. One provider's prevention strategy includes: specialized educational programs at the preschool and elementary levels to make learning more exciting and to broaden the intellectual horizons of children-at-risk; attitude change such that fatalism is discouraged and social activism is promoted; the nonreinforcement of these ailments by withholding disability payments; the active indoctrination of clients with the work ethic, such that they might be socially productive and adequately financially remunerated; and finally, active vocational training and rehabilitation programs. The value judgments implicit in these recommendations appear to be related to a view that people with nerves are "culturally deprived."

Among Costa Ricans *nervios* (nerves) is etiologically linked to family disruption and a breakdown in family relationships (Low, 1981). Here nerves provide a socially acceptable category of physical and mental disturbances for the symptoms of being "out of control" or separated from body and self. For some groups like Puerto Ricans, *nervios* may be a reason for consulting spiritists. Some Colombians relate it to debility, or consider it a woman's problem as do some Iranians. Some African Americans relate nerves to frustration and anger, family worries, too many responsibilities, lack of appreciation from and avoidance by family members, death, spouse abandonment or abuse, and poverty. Dizziness appears to be an analogous syndrome among some Asian clients. Nerves, and other cultural idioms of distress, appear to express to health practitioners, in a coded form, information which would otherwise be culturally inappropriate or difficult to present. Such community defined illness allows people to signal social "dis-ease" encoded through a culturally acceptable body disturbance (Low, 1981). Research suggests that the Western professionally defined role of patient is not the goal of the person expressing community-defined illness behavior, rather the intent is reconnection to the community.

An exploratory study of *nervios* among Puerto Rican women reported that it is more commonly found among women rather than men, and that it is etiologically linked to conflicted family relations (Wolf Dresp, 1985). The contemporary presentation of *nervios* differs from a past manifestation in that *nervios* now serves to secure aid from *outside* the family. This is related to the profound impact that social economic developments have had on the Puerto Rican family. Within the present day context of Puerto Rican life, *nervios* as a request for family aid that will serve to reintegrate the sufferer into the family system is ignored, unresponded to, or not recognized. Many Puerto Rican families are now "split," hence the traditional extended family and friends network is disrupted such that obligations to care are spread among fewer individuals, who themselves are already taxed. Since support from these individuals is not provided to *nervios* sufferers, *nervios* may serve to secure aid outside the family and may actually serve to separate individuals from the family.

Others report that some Puerto Ricans and Central Americans suffer from *ataques de nervios*, a pseudo-epileptic outburst of screaming or aggressiveness that at times includes pseudo-suicidal behavior (De La Cancela, Guarnaccia, & Carrillo, 1986). A critical analysis of such *ataques*, suggests that they serve social uses, are related to social economic status, and are socially learned. Depending on the setting an *ataque* can have different precipitants (e.g., loss, shock, conflictual situations). On a macro level *ataques* can serve as culturally sanctioned responses to colonization/oppression that allow expressions of repressed anger in a guilt-free manner and permit secondary gains. On a micro level they can be related to post-traumatic stress disorders and sexual or child abuse histories. From the intrapsychic perspective they can also allow for tension discharge that is ego integrative.

In concert the above provide clues as to how health practitioners should proceed when presented with the complaints of *nervios*. Practitioners should move discussion to personal and familial topics in a friendly nonthreatening way, inquiring about recent losses, problems with family members and friends, legal problems, chemical dependencies, or illness. Providers might also share their own similar topical experiences as a way of establishing rapport and framing inquiries. They should be careful to explain the rationale for their questions so as to not appear prying. As such, nerves may be understood not as the complaint of a difficult patient but as a positive help-seeking behavior attempting to reestablish a balanced socioemotional state. Though patients may request medication for the complaint, it may not be effective or helpful. Rather, supportive counseling or psychoeducation regarding social stressors and multidisciplinary team involvement may be more helpful to the patient.

Depression and Somatization

Somatization frequently expresses social as well as emotional distress, and at times it represents only social problems. Somatization is often a manifestation of depression, but is not restricted to depression. It can be a result of hypochondriasis, conversion disorders, or a socially learned way of communicating psychological distress. Depression often is expressed somatically by patients whose cultural labelling, reporting, or views minimize verbal expression of depression. Rather nonverbal means of communicating depression are socially and culturally acceptable and encouraged. Such patients may originate from sociocultural groups which include: fundamentalist religious groups; the less educated working class; and rural dwellers. The idea that depressed patients can perceive a dysphoric affective state and can report it to practitioners is a twentieth-century invention of Western culture where "psychological mindedness" is expected. Indeed many other cultures do not value and often stigmatize the expression and perception of emotions. In these cultures depression, connotes weakness, "craziness," moral culpability, and loss of face, while physical complaints are legitimate cues for obtaining nurturance, care, and sympathy. For instance, among the Chinese the linking of mind, body, and soul shapes the way in which depression is expressed. Chinese will describe heart palpitations, loss of appetite, sleeplessness, dizziness, and stomach aches as common somatic complaints. Such cultures may promote vegetative or somatic symptoms as a way to communicate and concretize emotions. Or, these states may be known by other terms, for instance, among some Latinos(as) there exists an illness called *susto* which includes weakness, decreased appetite, insomnia, motor retardation, and decreased libido. Yet this symptom constellation might be labeled as agitated depression by Western health practitioners. Some Asians report heart palpitations and dizziness as equal to anxiety, and stomach aches, decreased appetite and depression as correlates of chronic fatigue syndrome. For some older African Americans, depression and other psychological and physical disorders are simply referred to as "a bad spell" where one has little or no control. Among some North American males one may also see more somatic complaints, given gender socialization experiences that include being told "to take pain like a man."

Somatization related to psychological dynamics may also be used to control and manipulate family relationships; to avoid or take time out from stressful social situations like work, sex, and close relationships; to justify dependency; and to punish others. It may also be a result of practitioners preferentially looking for and treating somatic complaints and not monitoring the psychosocial aspects of the patient's illness. This last point reflects the perception of the practitioner as a support that is lacking in the rest of the patient's life whose attention, interest, and empathy can only be generated by somatic complaints. This may lead to circular cycles of more physical symptoms being reinforced by attention. Additionally, physical complaints have more positive connotations than emotional complaints in Western society as can be seen by the compensations and economic remuneration provided for physical disease (Katon, Kleinman, & Rosen, 1982).

Depression is a disorder that should be viewed from a psychocultural perspective because both its diagnosis and treatment are affected by such factors. For example, diagnostically the provider needs to ask: What is the cultural meaning of feeling drowsy or sedated, or of having sexual problems? How do both the failure to meet sex-role expectations *and* meeting them contribute to depression disorders? For example, among low income Latinos/as the male provider role is challenged by being un- or underemployed; among

Latina females ascribed child rearing roles, poverty, single parent-hood, and absent partners create stress; and among some African American women rejection in relationships often compounds preex-isting depression or emotional pain associated with varied psy-chosocial pressures and devaluation (De La Cancela, 1990b).

From a therapeutic perspective antidepressant medication com-pliance might be affected by sociocultural beliefs, values, and atti-tudes regarding fear of addiction, side effects, diet restrictions, and the stigma of conditions requiring medication. For example, if rela-tives or friends have had side effects from certain drugs or con-versely experienced benefits, the patient may choose not to take prescribed drugs or choose to ingest alternative home remedies. In addition, negligent and unethical management of psychotropic med-ication by some practitioners in communities of color have served as barriers to trust and compliance.

The health practitioner is therefore advised to avoid sanctioning indefinite periods of disability benefits for patients with somatic complaints; to encourage clients to view somatic complaints as their bodies' inherent way of communicating that they should take care of themselves for all is not right in their interpersonal or social spheres (Hilliard, 1980); to not simply reassure or be inattentive toward pa-tients; and to engage in specific questioning. Questions should be asked such as: Did you have a parent or sibling with a chronic ill-ness who received special care and attention? Is there other illness in your present family? How has this illness affected your family? Do your symptoms get worse under specific circumstances? What are those? (Rosen, Kleinman, & Katon, 1982)

Severe Mental Illness

The secondary features of mental illness, such as the content of delusions and hallucinations are influenced by cultural factors (Kiev, 1972). Once an individual is labelled as mentally ill, he is guided by a number of cultural cues which tell him how to play that role (Waxler, 1977). That is to say that the mentally ill person learns how to be sick in a way his/her particular society understands. In-deed, in many traditional societies members expect mental illness to be brief and easily cured; these beliefs are reinforced by the treat-ment system and the patient's family, hence patients mold their ex-periences to these expectations.

Western psychiatric diagnosis, for the most part, is based on the practitioner's subjective evaluation of the patient's appearance, speech, and behavior. Hence diagnoses are influenced by the personal, social, and cultural views of mainly medical practitioners, as well as diagnostic fashions and changing views of etiology. Psychiatric labeling can at times function to validate stereotypes in as much as diagnostic criteria is based on "aberrations" from the cultural norms. For example, the behavior of ethnic patients may be judged schizophrenic by Westerners, thereby suggesting that the culturally different are irrational and bizarre by medical standards. Since schizophrenia is apt to be primarily conceptualized as a medical illness, given the genetic evidence and clear-cut efficacy of phenothiazines for its treatment, psychopharmacology rather than social change is the suggested intervention (Lazare, 1973).

Thus, an ensuing tendency to overdiagnose and overmedicate can occur when the patient presents with *ataque de nervios* symptoms that appear similar to epileptic seizures or ethnospiritual beliefs as *espiritismo* among some Latinos/as or protective spirits among Asian subgroups that appear, to the culturally incompetent, equivalent to schizophrenia. Professional unfamiliarity with the culturally diverse and comparative biases can also contribute to the underdiagnosis of less severe or primitive mental illness such as depression among communities of color.

HEALTH CARE PRACTICES: NUTRITION

Each culture defines what is edible and what is not, such that food which is eaten in one society is forbidden in another. Culture also defines food such that some have assumed more symbolic value and less nutritional significance. Within the Asian culture, for example, chicken is used for both medicinal/health values and to celebrate festive occasions. Class defines foods in a manner that leads to certain foods having more or less "prestige value" (Farb & Armelagos, 1980; Helman, 1978). Additionally, many cultures use some foods for their soothing effects rather than nutritional value. When parents routinely soothe infants to sleep with milk, juice or sweetened water, the child's dental health can be negatively affected even prior to the appearance of the first teeth.

These practices may affect individuals in two ways: (a) they may exclude necessary nutrients from their diet and (b) they may encourage the consumption of certain foods which are harmful. When both conditions combine, there is a greater likelihood of poor nutrition and over-eating. Overeating, in particular, may lead to obesity and other disorders among African Americans, West Indians, Latino/as, and Asians who may view "big fat babies" as healthier than average weight children. This is important since obesity in childhood may lead to obesity in adulthood. Hence, practitioners should attend to their patient's dietary habits in order both to identify areas where they might be at risk of poor nutritional intake, and to intervene by recommending diets that are in line with cultural mores, when appropriate. Additionally, health care providers should be sensitive to the psychosocial aspects of malnutrition in a Western capitalist society. For example, it is possible that some poor families come to view malnutrition as their norm given their lower expectations of good health due to the lack of available medical, economic, and nutritional resources. Such families may also avoid the stigma of having its members diagnosed as having malnutrition in an affluent society that tends to blame poverty on its victims (Ryan, 1976).

EXPLANATORY MODELS: HEALTH BELIEFS

Patients may deny their illnesses or view them as related to personal carelessness or weakness, feelings of inadequacy or powerlessness, self-blame or punishment, or as external forces over which they have no control and are not responsible for. Practitioners may view the same illness as related to diet, genetics, or occupational hazards. Disease is what the practitioners objectively discover, while illness is what the patient subjectively experiences (Helman, 1981). Illness is the psychological experience of disease as defined by individual and community views of health. Different views about ill-health are often based on economic factors. An illustration is provided by working-class mothers who did not define themselves or their children as ill even when they had symptoms, since they continued to function socially or were able to carry on with activities of daily life (Helman, 1985). Sometimes the denial of illness is influenced by the necessity to continue working for as long as possible due to limited financial resources or extensive caretaking responsibilities. Denial can also stem from having difficulty with asking for help due to social conditioning. Hence, the cooperation of others is necessary before the patient can adopt the "sick role" and be defined as temporarily unable to fulfill social obligations to family, friends, or co-workers and become eligible for care by others. Etiological conceptualizations interact with other social economic factors like whether the patient can afford or has access to health care. Psychocultural factors include work being a primary source of self-esteem, and acknowledging and seeking health care as a form of self-caretaking that historically has not been permitted by the pressures that marginalized peoples endure. In concert, the basis for consulting practitioners includes: the failure or success of treatments within the popular/folk sectors (self-help groups, religious groups), the patient's perception of the problem, and how others perceive the problem (Zola, 1966).

As such, the decision to consult practitioners is often related to sociocultural factors rather than the severity of the illness. These factors may also affect treatment compliance. Furthermore, since patients may consult with others in their network (friends, family, neighbors) before they seek medical care and thereby select what is brought to health practitioners, it is possible that reported epidemiological differences between groups reflect such selective processes (Zola, 1966).

It is recommended that practitioners should treat both illness and disease in their patients at the same time, thereby attempting to restore the patient's health within her "supportive group—cognitive system network" (Alder & Hammett, 1973). Along these lines, culturally competent diagnostic practices should include:

1) stressing more informality and personalism in history taking (Rosado, 1980);
2) placing an increased emphasis on explanation, labeling, and validation;
3) responding to the personal, family, and community issues surrounding illness;
4) identifying and acknowledging social roles and social distance factors;
5) being respectful of and open to cultural differences even if these appear "strange" from the perspective of the practitioner.

Specific questions that practitioners can ask to discover the patient's "explanatory models" are offered in the following table.

TABLE 3.1

ILLNESS BELIEFS/HEALTH PRACTICES INQUIRY

Is there any specific time of the day the problem occurs?
What do you think it does to you?
How do family or others around you respond to the problem?
What activities lead to an increase or decrease in the problem?
What can you no longer do because of the problem?
What are the results you hope to receive from the treatment?
What are the problems your sickness has caused you?

(Adapted from Kleinman, 1980, and Brockway, 1980)

Patient response to the questions should be compared with practitioner's views openly, suggesting alternative views to the patient and attempting to explain them from the patient's point of view if their model will significantly interfere with appropriate care (Kleinman, et al., 1978). In this regard a harmful practice may be eliminated if it is suggested that since it has not seemed to work, something else may be tried (C.S. Scott, 1974). In essence, explanatory models must be negotiated to increase the patient's repertoire of health information and the practitioner's knowledge of appropriate intervention (Helman, 1985). The aim of the practitioner should be to reduce ambiguity for patients by compassionately providing information as to the nature, course and prognosis of their disease from a biopsychosocial perspective (Jospe, Nieberding, & Cohen, 1980).

CONCLUSION

The focus of this chapter has been on providing providers with a knowledge base, some skills and abilities, and attitudes that aid them in partnering with clients to answer the essential question of "How do you view health?" Therapeutic alliances require negotiation and clear communication of health status concepts, beliefs, and psychosocial and cultural information. As partners, clinician and consumer can explore how their health care orientations influence perception of health needs and consequently health status. The intersection of the popular, folk, and professional sectors' codes and rituals may impact whether a patient ever gains entry to the primary health care provider's consultation room. For example, Asian immigrants' knowledge of health care systems is limited by what is supplied by friends, family, and sponsors from within the community; the second and third generation Latino/a client's culturally based concepts of health care and practices may include reliance on folk medicine, fear of unfamiliar medical practices, and notions of proper decorum, modesty, reserve, and control of the expression of fear and pain; and the uninsured and poor African American male may feel helpless, inferior, and defeated when confronted with the inadequate resources available to meet the needs of the medically underserved.

Additionally, as a result of national and local change, communities of diversity are increasing in the United States, such that consumers from these groups both seek and expect systems of care that encourage self-sufficiency and cultural integrity, and provide linguistic options. Latino/as, African Americans, Asian Americans, Native Americans, gays, lesbians, women, psychiatric survivors, the physically challenged, and the elderly in this country have all developed a sense of empowerment over the past several decades of liberation movements, which makes them increasingly critical health consumers (Walker, 1994). The poor and underserved, communities of color, and other disenfranchised groups have increased awareness of how they have suffered impaired health status due to miscommunication, under-, over-, and misdiagnosis, culturally incompetent treatment, and lack of access to primary care. Culturally competent clinicians can meet the challenges of empowered consumers by attending to psychosocial stressors, differentiating between culturally acceptable behaviors and pathology, examining ethnoracial diversity in disease prevalence and reaction to medication, formulating treatment plans which are culturally appropriate, utilizing community resources, and respecting the adaptability and survival skills of patients (Walker, 1994).

Cultural competence also requires looking beyond the obvious dimensions of race, ethnicity, and culture to values and gender issues in individual health behaviors, health practice, health policy, and health research. Here the questions are: How do we as providers view health? How do we view men and women? What are the values of and views about ethnicity and gender which influence health behaviors? Are we to continue subscribing to reductionistic medical models or psychological approaches that consider gender and cultural differences as confounding results? Do we endanger people's health by ignoring difference? Do we contribute to the oppression, exploitation, or disenfranchisement of major sectors of our society by making health decisions for them or uncritically supporting practices deemed more beneficial to us or others than to the client? We need to review our professional contributions to socioeconomic issues and psychocultural factors that mitigate healthy behaviors. Do we support the use of Caesarian sections as convenient and predictable for physicians? Do we support tubal ligations and sterilization of "less desirable" populations, i.e., the mentally retarded or developmentally delayed, the substance abuser or mentally ill, ethnoracial groups with high birth rates, or the person with HIV or AIDS? Do we place obstacles to the consumer's exercise of her rights in accessing medical records or limit their informed consent to treatment by not providing information in developmentally and linguistically appropriate print and audio visual materials?

COMMENTARY

Jane S. Lin-Fu

In this book, the authors examine health in terms of health needs, health status and health care systems at the community level. They propose a community health psychology perspective that will help to bring about a better understanding of the psychosocial and cultural dimensions of health. This basic understanding is essential in any attempt to improve access to the health care delivery system. It is also indispensable in making services offered by the system more culturally relevant and appropriate for the target population. This expanded horizon and approach to health care is particularly important for communities of color which are often poorly served by a health care system that is still largely designed and administered by those in the mainstream of society. In Chapter Three, the authors explore the role of psychosocial and cultural factors in determining differential manifestations of health status and/or diagnosis in different ethnocultural groups. This is an important facet of health and health care that has been generally overlooked in the medical literature.

Until recently, the biomedical model used in the U.S. health care system has largely ignored the role of psychosocial and cultural factors in determining health beliefs, concepts, behavior, and ultimately, health status. The adverse outcome of this unidimensional approach has been particularly evident in communities of color, many of whom have been unable to gain access to the existing health care system. Even after gaining entry, many have not truly benefited from the services offered because such services have been psychosocially unacceptable, economically unaffordable, or culturally inappropriate or even offensive. It is therefore not surprising to find that many resources aimed at improving the health status of racial and ethnic minorities have been wasted through the delivery of unwanted and unresponsive services to communities that are outside or on the fringe of the United States mainstream. Despite much good intention and effort, and considerable expenditures, improvement in health status of racial and ethnic minorities in the United States has been less than impressive.

Recent dramatic changes in the U.S. health care system, including the rapid expansion of managed care, have been viewed by some as reaching crisis proportions. Turning to the Chinese language and philosophy, one finds the word "crisis" to be made up of two characters: "danger" and "opportunity." In short, every danger offers an opportunity. A crisis should therefore not be simply viewed negatively as a danger or threat, but rather positively, as an opportunity to bring about changes and improvements. As the U.S. health care system seeks to trim waste, improve cost-effectiveness of its health services and expand its coverage for an increasingly diverse population, those committed to equal access to effective health services for all should capture this opportunity to make the health care system truly responsive to all communities.

To bring about this desperately needed change in the health care system, it is critical for legislators, health care policymakers, planners, administrators and direct service providers to realize that health is a culturally-bound concept that has different meanings to persons of different backgrounds. As noted in Chapter Three, manifestation of diseases may be described and interpreted differently by different ethnic groups. The mode of help-seeking and method of communication between health service consumers and providers may also differ widely among diverse populations. Furthermore, patient expectations, satisfaction and compliance with prescribed treatment are all closely intertwined with one's cultural, psychosocial, and economic background. Unless the health care system makes a sincere and concerted effort to understand the nonbiomedical and nonmainstream dimensions of illnesses, especially in terms of health beliefs and behavior in communities of color, and makes the necessary adjustments to meet a community's need, it is highly questionable that the health services it offers can ever be effective or cost-effective with nonmainstream populations.

Lastly, in attempting to serve any *community, one must not lose sight of the fact that all persons should be considered as individuals first before they are viewed as part of a community. For communities of color, sensitivity and recognition of intra-ethnic variations as well as uniqueness of individual needs are keys to avoiding stereotyping—an offense that is deeply hurtful to racial and ethnic minorities. Beyond understanding the dynamics of psychosocial, economic, and cultural factors in a community, it is also crucial that the health care system prove itself to be worthy of trust of the community without which a sound ongoing relationship cannot be expected.*

Over the last three decades or so, racial and ethnic minorities have increased at a rate three times that of the total U.S. population. Today, one in every four persons in the U.S. is a racial or ethnic minority. The U.S. Census Bureau projects that by the year 2050, non-Hispanic Caucasians will make up only 52.7% and people of color will comprise nearly half of the U.S. population. The U.S. health care system no longer has the choice of ignoring the special health care needs of one quarter of its population, i.e., its communities of color. Any effort to improve the health care system for the nation can be successful only if it approaches health as a multidimensional issue and gives due consideration to the unique unmet needs of its diverse population.

SECTION II

APPROACHES TO CHANGE

Nancy J. Kennedy

The nation's health care system is undergoing rapid and dramatic change. In the current restructuring, managed care organizations (MCOs) have grown from a handful of small utilization review firms serving large corporate clients to a major industry that manages care for more than half of the nation's population. The excellence of the U.S. health care system, pontificated in certain sectors, is not ubiquitous within the fabric of this multicultural country. Research has consistently shown that many vulnerable populations receive disparate routine medical care and are disproportionately uninsured (Aday, 1993).

The significant impacts of the managed care industry are being experienced at both the micro- and the macro-level. As managed care systems grow and assume responsibility for larger segments of the population, especially those financed with public funds such as the recipients of Medicaid and Medicare, community-based approaches need to be a critical complement to individual clinical interventions. Population-based risk factor rating analyses, a more targeted method for MCOs, could potentially reduce not only high health care costs but also improve access and consumer satisfaction.

The explosiveness of managed care has created confusion and uncertainty not only for health care organizations but also for individuals, including health care professionals, consumers, and family members. At present, critical decisions are the purview of politicians and purchasers. Medical care providers are quickly beginning to mobilize and form competing networks. Unfortunately, most consumers, family members, advocates, and community health providers are on the periphery of the evolution of managed care.

Their lack of involvement and that of their current community-based providers are noticeably absent in the planning and proposed implementation of state Medicaid waivers and other managed care contracts.

States, as companies have done for several decades in the private sector, are contracting with MCOs to provide health care services (Scheffler & Radany, 1990). Although the tendency has been for states to contract with profit-making MCOs, those organizations have relatively little experience providing public sector services. MCOs are required, both with the accreditation process and in fulfilling contractual parameters, to be responsive to community demographics and to the cultural needs of the populations that they serve. Some states and/or MCOs have contracts or subcontracts with community-based organizations (CBOs) whose cultural morés are more characteristic of the target population(s). These CBOs recognize both the risks and opportunities in working with MCOs. Nonetheless, these public-private partnerships can result in achieving empowered communities that are able to acquire mastery for themselves and all the citizenry (Wolff, n.d.)

Empowerment "brings diverse people to an understanding of themselves as members of a specific sub-population and allow(s) them to gain access to others with similar social identity" (Luna & Rotheram-Borus, 1995). Empowerment can occur at both the macro- and micro-level. Like other situations, the turbulent changes in the health care system have exacerbated feelings of frustration, powerlessness, and disenfranchisement. Of all health consumers, those most at risk are people who are economically and socially disadvantaged. The situation could easily worsen as welfare reform evolves and becomes intertwined with health care reform. In addition, given this country's recent rapid growth through immigration and a high birth rate due to the youthfulness of many immigrants, many people of color groups will, in the next century, no longer be labeled "minority" populations. Hence, the cultural proficiencies of organizations will enhance their sustainability into the next millennium.

Change is not an easy process, especially if the goal is empowerment; but cognition, beliefs, values, needs, attitudes, and experiences can be transformed and community health psychology is primed to accomplish the necessary changes. For example, the informational element of informed consent is one leverage that health consumers have in becoming empowered at the micro-level. At the macro-level, encouraging the participation of MCOs with CBOs in designing and implementing behavioral health promotion and disease prevention strategies can significantly decrease health care costs since most of today's morbidity and mortality are associated with diseases of lifestyle.

Decades of public sector experience in consumer and family empowerment strategies in the mental health field have produced replicable models such as consumer self-help, case management, family advocacy, community-based alternatives to hospitalization, social rehabilitation, residential programs, and half-way houses. These models can demonstrate significant cost savings while engendering empowerment and increased quality of life. In addition, the intentional design and implementation of culturally accessible, responsive, and competent services hold the potential for increasing member retention and customer satisfaction.

Encouraging the development of health programs and disease management strategies can also shift responsibility for health care from providers to consumers. Placing the onus for health and well-being back into the hands of the people should increase more direct responsibility of health care status and, ultimately, reduce the demand for services utilization. At the present time, people view most illnesses (including behavioral disorders) as something beyond their control. The role of patients with behavioral disorders can easily be characterized as a passive, sometimes negative role, which when accompanied by cultural stigma strips people of even their dignity, and results in negative verbalizations against the providers and systems whose true aim is to help.

There exist extraordinary opportunities within this changing health care environment. "Health promotion is (or should be) characterized by efforts to link actions at different social levels in some coherent way" (Labonte, 1994). Vigorous well-designed programs of health promotion and disease prevention require active participation which can affect in a positive manner all aspects of the system transforming it from sickness care to health care. Assertive leadership is critical; as visionaries, the planners of a community-oriented primary care system (Starfield, 1992) must either be ahead of or riding the wave of change or they will suffer the devastation of the flood.

4

Community-Oriented Health Service Delivery: A Systemic Approach

Jean Lau Chin, Victor De La Cancela,
and Yvonne M. Jenkins

The parallel rise of community health centers and community mental health centers in the 1970s led to a new paradigm in health care service delivery systems to serve the poor and medically underserved (Patton, 1990; Plaska & Vieth, 1995; Rosenbaum, 1987). It was a departure from a focus on the individual patient toward a focus on the needs of communities. It was also an application of public health concepts to prevent, treat, and rehabilitate, i.e., to meet unmet needs. Furthermore, it included the community and the people within that community as a context—the health of a community. The emergence of this movement highlighted the importance of a systemic approach to health care and the value of community based systems of care. The importance of advocacy within political and social contexts, and an attention to the influence of policy on our service delivery systems became an integral part of discussions on health care. More important, the movement fused the separation between public and private sectors as community-based agencies played very public roles in the delivery of health and mental health care.

THE PARADOX OF THE COMMUNITY HEALTH AND MENTAL HEALTH MOVEMENTS

Contemporaneously when the integrity of community-based systems are threatened by cost containment reform measures, we are underscoring the importance of infrastructures needed to sustain these systems. To understand the elements of the community health and mental health center movements, we need to understand the dyadic tensions within the field from which it grew. The inadequacies of a purely biomedical model in the health sector gave rise to biopsychosocial practices in community health centers (Overall & Williamson, 1988; Wertlieb, 1979) while the inadequacies of a clinical psychopathology model in the mental health sector gave rise to hybrid clinical-community psychology practices in community mental health centers (Iscoe, 1974). These practices were attempts to address those sociocultural and cultural problems which could not be solved within the context of the individual patient-doctor relationship or clinical visit. Poverty, lack of insurance, social problems, cultural unfamiliarity, and learned inability to negotiate the health care delivery system were deterrents to utilization and influenced adverse health outcomes.

Initially, this meant perhaps little more than providers connecting with the community and being sensitive to their needs. The imperative to alter "traditional" or "standard" service delivery practices soon became evident as client practices and beliefs influenced compliance. Case management, community education, and outreach were necessary to promote access to care. The importance of advocating for patient needs grew as the barriers of language, culture, or poverty faced by clients became evident. Policy, regulatory, and systemic changes were necessary to insure viability of care and access to services within the macro system of which community health centers were a part. In short, we began to pay attention to the social, community, familial, political, public health, and macro system contexts influencing the delivery of health and mental health services.

The community health movement occurred in the context of the civil rights movement of the 1960s in which the call to action by President John F. Kennedy represented the idealism of the time to serve, and give back, to the community. It was part of the war on poverty and racism. This movement also emphasized community-based services and community organizing. This era was quickly followed by the 70s, the Vietnam War, disillusionment with the "Great Society," and the pessimism of the 1970s. The "me generation" of the 1980s emphasized an egocentricity within the mental health field evidenced by an emphasis on developing theories of self-psychology and private practice over community service in the career goals of professionals entering the field. The proliferation of free clinics founded in the 1960s began its decline (Free Clinic Foundation, 1990). As the emphasis on technology and specialty care grew, so did our health care costs and emphasis on risk management. The 1990s saw the emphasis on cost containment, growth of managed care, and discussions on the rationing of health care. These sociopolitical contexts undoubtedly influenced the developments within our health and mental health service delivery systems.

While similar changes in our community health and mental health systems occurred, these systems interacted little in providing care. They remained separate and distinct as though behavioral and psychological factors had no influence on physical health and well-being. Yet, their principles of care instructed and influenced one another. While psychology initially imitated medicine's diagnostic and curative perspective to treatment, medicine began to recognize the importance of psychological phenomena and its impact on health care and utilization. It became evident that a person-oriented approach over a disease-oriented one could positively influence compliance and outcomes (DiMatteo & Tarenta, 1979). Lifestyle behaviors (smoking, diet, exercise) correlated with disease and health status. More awareness of how social and environmental conditions (lead poisoning, pollution, and toxic wastes) influenced adverse health outcomes also developed.

Community health centers have been important as a model for serving the medically underserved and currently meet the medical needs of 8.8 million people through 850 health centers nationwide (National Association of Community Health Centers [NACHC], 1995); still, regulations and policies governing these centers often fail to include all segments of the population. Positive as the growth of community health and mental health centers has been, disenfranchised communities of color continue to experience a disproportionate share of negative health outcomes (Heckler, 1985; The Commonwealth Fund, 1995). The macro system continues to pose barriers such that persons of color do not have full access to the U.S. health care service delivery system. Systems of care designed for specific ethnic communities are marginalized as inferior, transitional, or unessential. As we now know, poverty persists disproportionately among our communities of color (Boston Persistent Poverty Project, 1989; Sagara & Kiang, 1992) and correlates with negative health status and access to care. There is a new war on poverty in response to the failure of social welfare policies as communities of color remain disproportionately underserved.

In communities where language and culture pose significant problems in accessing health care, the impact of poverty heightens the inadequacies within our macro systems of care. As a case in point, South Cove Community Health Center is located in Boston's

Chinatown, a small geographic area densely concentrated with physicians given its urban location near major academic teaching centers. Chinatown is viewed as community to many Asian Americans who live in greater Boston outside the immediate geographic area. While South Cove was successful in getting the Asian population designated as a Medically Underserved Population (MUP), and Chinatown as a Health Professional Shortage Area (HPSA) based on the language and cultural needs of the immigrant and refugee population in the 1970s, it has faced significant barriers as these MUPs and HPSAs come up for redesignation. Because these designations focus on an ethnic population, it remains an exception and secondary to designations based on geography. Whereas these federal designations are intended to target poverty areas, they become eligibility criteria for federal community health center funding and recruitment of National Health Service Corp (NHSC) physicians. The priority given to geographic designations has been inflexible in meeting ethnic population needs.

When funding was available to expand community health centers in 1993 for the first time in 10 years, emphasis was given to community health centers expanding within their service areas. Asian community health centers, which had been level funded for over a decade despite the tripling of the Asian population, were generally ineligible to expand their services to the Asian population because their population focus would result in their crossing over into other service areas. Similarly, in the redesignation of HPSAs, it was necessary first to demonstrate that the geographic area did not meet the criteria for a shortage of physicians serving low income populations before one could apply for a designation based on a shortage of bilingual physicians serving the Asian population. While these regulations and policies made "logical" sense in "simplifying the process" of redesignation, they resulted in a cumbersome, extraordinary, and duplicative process for those community health centers targeting specific ethnic/linguistic communities of color. Moreover, the National Health Service Corps, intended to increase the supply of physicians to medically underserved areas, has given no priority to the recruitment of bilingual candidates needed to work with immigrant and refugee communities. When qualified candidates are identified by community health centers through their own recruitment strategies, it is generally not possible to get them designated for NHSC slots. While the example is specific to the Asian community, it reflects the scenario for communities which come together based on ethnic/linguistic affiliation over that of geographic proximity.

Dyadic Perspectives

Within this context, a community-oriented health psychology perspective captures multiple dialectics. These tensions can be useful in moving the field toward models which promote the health of all our communities. Paradigm shifts are needed to ensure that the premises upon which community health center models are based remain loyal to the mission of serving all underserved segments of the population. Using community as the unit of intervention, this systemic approach captures the dyad of "macro system vs. community perspectives" in our delivery of health care. At the community level, community-based and community-sensitive practice can instruct and inform our macro system of care without losing sight of the individual. Where the U.S. macro system has promoted expensive technology and specialty care as a unit of intervention, it has not been informed and modified by the specific needs and practices (as dictated by culture, ethnicity, income level, language, history) of specific communities. An approach which joins this dyad through its advocacy and policymaking will reduce adverse outcomes and barriers to care. A second dyadic perspective of "administrator vs. provider" reflects the policy and practice roles needed to instruct and influence one another. Administrator and provider need to interact from a systemic, community-oriented perspective to examine differences in the health beliefs and health status of a community while avoiding the pitfalls of victim blaming. In this sense, we capture a third dyadic tension of "policymaker vs. advocate." Within a community-oriented health service delivery system, these roles and its boundaries can be synthesized as providers represent both public and private sectors within a community health care system, play roles as both advocates and policymakers, and identify with both community and the macro system as members and providers. Within this community oriented health service delivery system, community empowerment and community competence remain important. A paradigm shift must focus on the needs of communities, not on artificial designations of neighborhoods and geographic areas determined by census tract data.

While notions of community empowerment and community competence are not new (Barbarin, Good, Pharr, & Siskind, 1981), they are placed in the conservative context (Jennings, 1994) of the 1990s. Retaliations against affirmative action are reflected in attempts to eliminate quotas and set asides despite continued disparities among communities of color. Anti-immigrant sentiment reflected in California's Proposition 187 to deny access to illegal immigrants has gained national momentum and expanded to deny benefits to legal immigrants as well. Social, welfare, and health care reform dominate the climate with their emphasis on cost containment, managed competition, and mega-systems to manage care. In this context, we need to be clear what we mean by communities, and develop systems of care which empower all communities, including communities of color.

Within this context, increased pressure for culturally competent systems of care has not necessarily led to increased access, but rather decreased resources for those systems that have historically provided community-based and ethnic specific care. We need to reframe the health care debate as both a civil rights and ethical issue (Chin, 1992). We need to be sensitive to and achieve competence with social and cultural issues as the diversity within the United States increases. Helpseeking behavior, the family as a player in the making of health care decisions, the disclosure of personal information within the physician-patient relationship, and the expression of emotion and perception of stress all are impacted by ethnocultural factors and need to be integrated into health care practices (Barker, 1992). The paradigm shift focuses on the contexts in which we live and the biases which we hold to move us toward models which support our recognition and respect for differences, and toward flexibility in our regulations and policies to enable communities whose differences do not reflect the majority to have their needs met competently.

Positive as the community health and mental health movement has been, few centers in the country have both health and mental health services integrated in a community service setting. Even fewer have social health components, which may indicate a failure to appreciate the necessity for this aspect of health at both group and individual levels. Despite the growing recognition that health and mental health are significantly interrelated, these systems of care have generally remained separate.

Developmental Perspectives and Psychological Principles

A community-oriented health psychology perspective also applies psychological principles of analysis to our systems of care. The influence of behavioral and psychological phenomena on adverse health outcomes and access to health care can serve to educate and guide us. The failure of smokers to heed warnings regarding the risks of smoking is a case in point (Elders, Perry, Eriksen, & Giovino, 1994; USDHHS, 1991). That psychology and medicine paradoxically interact as distant cousins reflects a tension and separation in our systems of care and a failure to reflect on organized health care belief systems about who is to be served, and how it should happen. Health care settings are dominated by a culture and organizational structure that are inconsistent with adequate psychosocial care (Tefft & Simeonsson, 1979).

Using psychological principles of analysis, developmental principles are important to understand the factors leading to change, growth, and adaptation in our systems of care. The individuals we treat, the communities we serve, and our systems of care are fluid and subject to developmental changes. Secondly, cycles of growth are important to understand the interaction of systemic and contextual factors with our systems of care. The interaction of the civil rights movement with the community health movement is a case in point. Third, the language used to describe our policy and practice is important in reflecting the biases and assumptions we make in our delivery of health care. Whether we define compliance or decision making as the choice made by our patients is crucial. Finally, the relationships inherent in our system of care between policymaker and community advocate, community and macro system, provider and patient roles include notions of authority, power and powerlessness, oppression and empowerment.

Ultimately, we are describing how a community health psychology perspective can promote the health of our communities. However, the inclusion of communities of color in this paradigm raises the question of how issues of diversity are addressed. Whereas communities of color are disproportionately located in urban areas, and whereas they are still a minority in most geographic areas of this country, paradigms which presume community to represent the mean of a group are artificial and irrelevant in meeting the specific needs of diverse communities. Moreover, paradigms which define access to care based on geographic definitions of community are likely to ignore the differences and diversity of our diverse communities. Consequently, the dyad between advocacy as a means of change and influence, and policymaking as a means of exercising responsible and accountable authority and power must ensure the participation of all voices. The paradigm defines a shift from the current macro system vis-a-vis the community, not unlike that of adult to child, to move toward a peer-to-peer relationship in the sharing of power. As such, the paradigm shifts toward a "mutually" valued relationship.

A new role for diverse communities within the U.S. macro system of care is one in which "we do with" rather than "have done to" as it has been in the past. We must look to a community health psychology perspective to re-engineer the role of health care policymakers and administrators and the significance of psychological concepts in our health care delivery system to promote community empowerment and community competence.

HEALTH REFORM: POLICY AND PRACTICE

In the mid-1990s, the urgency of rising health care costs resulted in reform measures toward cost containment, privatization, and managed care in the U.S. health care delivery system. These emergent issues call for reorienting of roles and rapid change. There has been an ambivalence in expectations of health reform and provision of health care. On the one hand, the emphasis on rugged individualism in the United States suggests that individuals take care of themselves, while the emphasis on generosity and compassion of our social ethic suggests that we take care of those unable to provide for themselves—access to health care is a basic right (Frank & Vandenbos, 1994). The United States has endorsed a wide range of goals, ranging from reduction of waste and inefficiency in health care costs to increased emphasis on prevention and providing coverage to the uninsured. This broad spectrum reflects how the beliefs and values of this society shape today's health reform debate (Blendon et al., 1994).

With the excitement of health care reform waxing and waning at the federal level, many agree that the states will play a key role in financing health care. Although President Clinton's Health Security Act put forward in 1993 was disregarded, it served as a catalyst for reform of the purchasing and delivery of health services. These proposals have ranged from comprehensive measures providing universal coverage to incremental proposals (Frank, Sullivan, & DeLeon, 1994). State initiatives have included: expanding financial access through taxes and employer mandates, controlling costs, improving delivery systems, and naming commissions to recommend future health reform legislation. Cost control measures have included market-driven approaches: health alliances and health insurance purchasing coalitions (HIPCs) offering consumer choice based on standard benefit packages to increase the purchasing power of small businesses; regulatory approaches, (e.g., play-or-pay initiative in Massachusetts); integrated service networks requiring responsibility for the health status of the community in which the system is located, thereby extending health system networks into underserved areas, often shifting financial risk from insurance companies to provider organizations. Through these discussions, several issues stand out as they impact culturally diverse communities.

FINANCING HEALTH CARE

Financing health care has been an important part of the debates on health care reform. One proposal has been employer mandates to pay 80% of the insurance premium, with the remainder paid by the employee. Subsidies would be provided to low-income individuals and low-wage firms. Given the higher frequency of small businesses and the higher uninsured rates within segments of communities of color, such an option is likely to disproportionately impact communities of color. This option might also result in businesses purchasing the cheapest health plan whether or not its benefits are adequate for its employees. Fixed, formula-based spending limits/caps, another option proposed, could preclude services for diseases more prevalent in specific communities of color (e.g., hepatitis B vaccination for Asian populations, treatment for sickle cell anemia in populations of African ancestry). Unfortunately, the discussion of financing has generally used price alone as the standard. Without an inclusion of discussions which protect basic principles of cultural competence, and promote the health of our communities, any financing option is likely to deny access to specific segments of the population; communities of color are likely to experience their disproportionate share.

Health Insurance

Universal health insurance coverage efforts for all U.S. residents to have access to care have met with significant opposition. The rate of uninsured among communities of color is disproportionate with 40% or greater compared to 14% in the general population.

Increasingly, fee for service health insurance plans are being replaced by managed care plans in the interest of cost containment. The incentives of a capitated fee under managed care plans, intended to contain costs and manage overutilization, are often a disincentive to utilization. In practice, it can work against the premise of a community-oriented approach which seeks to promote preventive care and early entry to care. The limiting of provider panels in order to control costs often has the net effect of limiting choice because criteria for linguistic and cultural competence are often not included in certifying providers.

Access to Care

Universal coverage should not be confused with universal access. Insurance coverage would not ensure the range of essential services for specific ethnic/racial groups. For example, few requirements exist for states to mandate translation/interpreter services or control quality and training of interpreters. Services necessary to ensure access to care, such as outreach, health education, case management, interpreter services, and social services, are not reimbursable, and therefore, not provided. Consequently, even those with health insurance coverage may not receive linguistically appropriate and culturally competent services.

INTEGRATED SERVICE NETWORKS

Shift Toward Primary Care

While the wonders of technology drove our systems of care toward increased specialization, its high costs with questionable benefits drove policymakers to rethink their necessity and cost effectiveness. A back-to-basics approach in medical care has shifted priorities back to primary care providers. Emphasis is now on integrated service networks to manage and maintain continuity of care. Less government is inherent in efforts to privatize and contract to mega-providers who can coordinate care and ration resources. Missing, however, is discussion as to whether any of these reform measures will improve the public's health (Feingold, 1994; Navarro, 1994). Generally absent in the debate on health care is how public health *must* emphasize social, behavioral, and environmental risk factors to health status, and how diverse communities can be integrated into this new and evolving context.

Essential Community Providers

Forces within the U.S. macro system over the past decade have resulted in an oversupply of specialists and an undersupply of primary care physicians. With the shifting emphasis on primary care training, funding for graduate medical education is now under review. Proposals have included creating a separate national fund from government and private insurers to pay for postgraduate medical education. Also proposed have been special payments to academic medical centers from a national pool of funds to support special costs associated with research, development of new medical technology and treatment of rare and unusually severe illnesses. Little discussion has included how these proposals will influence or be responsive to the needs of specific racial communities. For example, the existing pool of Asian physicians is often not bilingual, not primary care oriented, and/or does not choose to work with low income, non-English speaking Asian communities. The establishment of policy and practice priorities must exist to direct resources to meet unmet and emerging community needs, and to preserve existing community-based systems and community providers as we reevaluate our graduate medical training.

Integrated Service Networks

Integrated service networks are increasingly viewed as ways in which to coordinate care and contain costs within an environment of reform. These networks amount to mega-systems, i.e., large systems over wide geographic areas attempting to provide care for more persons. They are not community based. These networks involve the coordination, affiliation, and "partnership" between insurers, hospitals, physician practices, community health centers, and nursing homes. Variations have included the notion of regional health alliances which are large state or regionally based purchasing cooperatives set up to offer a choice of health insurance plans. With this emphasis on regional and integrated service networks, geographic boundaries have become a major criteria for defining services and access to care. Consequently, the needs among diverse communities, especially those with specific language, social, and cultural needs, will be overlooked as these networks are formed.

Using the Asian American population as an example, it is unlikely that plan benefits will meet their specific needs given that they make up less than 5% of the population in most neighborhoods, towns, and counties; emphasis of benefits will reflect the needs of the non-Asian majority population residing within that geographic area. Unfortunately, this is likely to replicate the barrier experienced by Boston's Chinatown discussed earlier, which had historically been subsumed under one of three different neighborhoods rather than self-defined as an ethnic community, thereby skewing any health data in the direction of indicators for that neighborhood. Consequently, the health needs of the Asian community remained undocumented and insignificant when masked by the dominant needs of the geographic area. For communities which define themselves by race and/or ethnicity over the geographic area in which they reside, the inflexibility of criteria and the use of a majority group to define the essential benefits will result in ignoring the specific needs and relevant services of diverse communities; these communities will then need to pay for needed services at additional costs.

Simultaneous with the development of regional or integrated service networks in obtaining insurance coverage is an increased emphasis on integrating systems of care. With the spread of managed care plans, the coordination and continuity of care from primary care to tertiary care settings takes on increased significance. Case management becomes more important as the primary care practitioner plays the role of gatekeeper in referring patients for specialty and tertiary health care. Low-income families, immigrant and refugee families, and diverse communities unfamiliar with the health care system, could be alienated further in a system with added regulations and authorization procedures necessary to access care. However, these families and communities will now become attractive to insurance plans because they represent potential enrollees who are low users of the system.

The development of collaborative partnerships between hospitals and community providers has flourished as hospitals now need to depend on primary care and community providers to refer patients. These have included joint ventures, joint physician practices, sharing property and staff, and collaborating on residency training. As these mega-systems develop, how and if they remain responsive to disenfranchised communities will be a challenge. We need to begin to redefine these networks to be responsive to diverse communities.

SOLUTIONS TO HEALTH REFORM: COMMUNITY-ORIENTED HEALTH CARE

Gaps within the U.S. health care system dovetailed with the sociocultural activism resulting in the community health and mental health movement of the 1960s. In the 1990s, cost containment provides the context for reform amidst the growing diversity of the United States population. A community health psychology perspective emphasizing the community as the unit of intervention and psychological principles as the units of analysis can provide a framework to guide us in this era of reform. Dyadic tensions should reflect a social responsibility to address the diversity of needs among communities of color and to meet the unmet needs among all segments of the U.S. population. Our solutions must empower communities. The competency of the macro system must be measured not only by measures of technology and cost savings, but also by measures of its effectiveness and cultural competence in promoting the health of diverse communities. Psychological principles can be used to examine, evaluate, and plan as the macro system interacts with community systems, and as policymakers dialogue with community advocates in ways which do not create new barriers. Instead, dialogue guided by such principles may eliminate those historic ones which have ignored the realities of marginalized diverse communities.

Instead of looking at health disparities under existing models, we must look at the health of a community defined by its members rather than convenient geographic areas or census tracts. Instead of focusing solely on underserved needs, we must explore how our systems can empower. Instead of descriptively examining the barriers, we must propose a system which promotes access. Our community health psychology approach needs to be inclusive of diverse communities. It needs to empower communities to ensure full access to care. It needs to be culturally competent to permit differential approaches for different groups. It needs to be systemic so that individuals are treated in their biopsychosocial, community, economic, family, and cultural contexts. Finally, it needs to be comprehensive so that preventive, primary, and tertiary care are coordinated.

In using this perspective to guide us toward solutions during an era of reform, we can frame three questions: 1) Who provides the care? 2) How does the health plan meet the needs of our diverse communities? 3) What policies and administrative structures govern the delivery of care and allocation of resources? As integrated service networks become increasingly viewed as the new way to coordinate care and contain costs within an environment of reform, we need to examine their ability to be culturally competent and empower diverse communities to improve access to care and health status in the United States. This will be illustrated through examples from an Asian, Latino/a, and African American perspective.

Community Health Network: Who provides the care?

When we examine the question of who provides the care, we must also examine the academic training and continuing education of providers to ensure that they remain committed to preserving community-based systems and training community providers who can practice in ways which target the health of a community. This can be done only if theories, courses, and field experiences expose students and professionals to these issues and provide frameworks for examining practice and health questions important to community health.

At the service level, we need to maintain and sustain the role of community providers and the role of community health centers in serving low-income, underserved populations. This can only be done with support for infrastructures which enables these systems to be sustaining. As cost cutting measures prevail, too often there is a piecemeal and fragmented approach to the reimbursement and funding of services. For example, funding of interpreter services on a piecemeal basis merely impacts its quality and prevents the development of systems which can coordinate these services more efficiently and realize cost savings.

As providers are increasingly organized by networks, what provider networks are there to ensure a comprehensive range of appropriate services for specific linguistic/ethnic communities? Representational or multicultural networks may not be sufficient to evaluate cultural competence.

Health Plan for the Community:
How does it meet the needs of the community?

As the pressure for reform drives changes to our existing system, managed care systems have grown in their share of the market. As transition periods for enrollment have occurred, many have been short and insensitive to the need to reach non-English–speaking populations. Health plans may not recognize or permit enrollment and coverage based on a consumer's definition of her community. For example, geographic access is but one of the variables consumers will use to choose where they get care. Restrictions which prevent choices or create barriers in making choices such as ethnic-specific services are unresponsive.

Employer mandates have been proposed where employers would pay 80% of the premium and employees would pay the remainder as a way to finance coverage. In communities with high uninsured rates, and greater dependency on small business, conversion is likely to have a disproportionate impact on communities of color. Employers and subscribers unaccustomed to paying insurance premiums are likely to choose on the basis of price over the availability of benefits without recognizing the impact until they need the services. Will there still be segments who are uninsured? Will their use of the health system result in higher costs than if we were to address their needs?

How are the gaps in services to be covered? Given the high use of alternative medicine among many communities of color (e.g., acupuncture and herbal medicine within Asian communities), the question of whether covering these services could result in cost savings to other services is a consideration. Given the disparities in health status among communities of color, standard benefits packages may not include coverage for specific services more important to the health of the community.

How do we maintain a focus on preventive programs and enabling services (e.g., interpreter support, case management, outreach, family planning, immunization, health education) necessary to ensure early entry and greater cost savings over the long term? The continued support of federal programs for these services may be a necessary component of any reform measure since the reimbursement system might not and should not cover all these services, and there will remain segments of the population who are uninsured.

Administrative and Governance Structures of a Network: What policies govern the delivery of care and allocation of resources?

The policies and administrative structures governing the delivery of care need to reflect the interests of all communities. Are communities of color included in the development and management of the system? Emphasis on geographic boundaries and regional networks being proposed in the insurance purchasing alliances could ignore the needs of specific communities if their numbers are insufficient to be represented and served by these broad alliances. Policies and administrative structures need to provide assurances that they will be responsive to these needs, ensure input and monitoring of plan options, and provide recourse for when they do not.

Fixed, formula-based spending limits/caps, for example, might preclude services which are needed primarily for specific populations. Therefore, how will the plan evaluate when certain groups are not receiving the care they need? What protection or sanctions will there be to ensure corrective action? What assurances are there that contract choices made by the state or employers will concur with patient and community choice and ensure reimbursement for needed services?

SERVICE NETWORKS FOR THE COMMUNITY: AN ASIAN AMERICAN EXAMPLE

How can a health network serve the needs of diverse communities? If it serves well the specific needs of a minority community, it has the potential to serve well the varied needs of the population at large. Using the Asian American community as an example, their definition as a community often includes multiple ethnicities, multiple languages and dialects while also making up only 3% of the population in most areas of the country. A single interpreter will not ensure culturally competent services when there are multiple languages and dialects spoken. Specific health beliefs, values, and practices may reduce medical compliance, outcomes, and utilization. Given the high prevalence of hepatitis B among Asian Americans, is it used as a health indicator, and is universal immunization covered as a standard benefit? Does the standard benefits package include the range of services specific to the health risks and disease status of the community (immigrants and refugees, low-income groups)? Or will these options be more costly to the community among which there are already high rates of uninsured? Are there limits to choice in choosing a provider under a managed care option? For example, will linguistic and cultural groups be forced to choose options which do not meet their needs? How does the plan ensure the highest quality of care, including linguistically appropriate and culturally competent care, at all points of patient contact? How does the plan ensure choice of plans or providers with appropriate linguistic capacity in their primary language? Is there flexibility in the plan to address the needs of Asians who are geographically dispersed, and generally do not constitute a majority even in areas where they are concentrated? Do regulations force designations of the Asian American population by census tracts or catchment areas, which would make their voices underrepresented in the allocation of resources and planning of priorities? Once the plan is chosen, how will administrative hassles be minimized, especially for non-English–speaking groups?

These questions speak to the importance of principles needed to guide and develop criteria for evaluating a health plan. They speak to the importance of diverse solutions, and ethnic-specific integrated service networks to ensure competency of the macro system in dealing with all segments of a diverse population.

Two sets of principles developed by the California Pan-Ethnic Health Network for health care reform (California Pan-Ethnic Health Network, 1992), and Boston At Risk 2000 (Boston at Risk 2000, 1994) emphasize the importance of communities and their self-determination in the development of a responsive health care system. They include as essential elements:

1) Health care as a human right
2) Elimination of individual and institutional racism
3) Language access at all points of patient contact
4) Representative governance
5) Participation by diverse communities at all levels
6) Cultural competency required at all levels
7) Necessity of cost containment
8) Mechanisms for community accountability
9) Preserve and promote community models of care
10) Prevention

SERVICE NETWORKS FOR THE COMMUNITY: A LATINO/A EXAMPLE

Having used networks in mental health policy, planning, training, consultation, advocacy, and curriculum, the second author recommends applying the model to urban Latino/a health policy reform. Formal introduction into the network model occurred in 1979 as fieldwork supervisor for Boston City Hospital's Minority Training Program (MTP) in Psychology, as a staff psychologist of the Hispanic Family Counseling Program at Massachusetts Mental Health Center, and expanding in 1980 as team leader of the Hispanic Outreach Team (HOT) of the Judge Baker Guidance Center in Boston. MTP and HOT shared a commitment to serving Boston's racially and ethnically diverse poor and working class populations. Each program utilized a network of similar minded clinicians to mobilize resources collectively, as many would have been prohibitively expensive to provide independently while carrying out agency specific missions of training or service delivery. In its simplest form, the network consisted of numerous voluntary members who were interested in advocacy, cultural activism, health and political education, and the development of alliances and coalitions to overcome institutional obstacles to accessing human services, (e.g., institutional racism).

The Hispanic Family Counseling Program and HOT were unique in their collaborative inclusion of health, mental health, and social services professionals along with community and indigenous workers to empower low income and underserved Latino/a individuals and communities. This perspective was a result of clinical-community psychology and public health orientation of both programs and a commitment to social activism among network members.

The intracultural and ethnic diversity of the network members and of the Latino/a populations served often led to programmatic interests in international public health models and political developments in Latino countries. Thus, the organization of health care delivery in Cuba, the empowerment pedagogy of Paulo Freire in Brazil, and the national liberation, decolonization, and anti-imperialist movements of the Americas were influential in shaping a commitment to therapeutic praxis and social reparation which can be called "terapia comprometida"—a therapy where there is a "bond of commitment," where the political, social, and psychological alliance between therapist and client is explicit (Becker, Lira, & Castillo, 1990).

Such therapeutic practice involves an ethically non-neutral attitude toward the client's problems, which is a conscious violation of the neutral stance advocated by mainstream psychotherapy. In the praxis of HOT and the Hispanic Family Counseling Program, being comprometido (committed) fostered the development of solidarity with the client and Latino/a community in their struggles against recurrent stress and trauma related to "differentness" in an intolerant society. Hence, client and mental health worker ideally entered into a relationship of compañerismo or therapeutic solidarity, that advocated for social justice, human rights, and access to quality health and human services (De La Cancela, 1995a).

Compañerismo reflects a sense of connection and responsibility which others within their specific racial and cultural contexts may label as Africanity or the Jungian collective unconscious (K. Crawford, personal communication). In the context of Native American, African, Asian, and Latino/a traditions and the experiences of people of color with oppression, it encourages partnerships and networking to meet survival challenges.

Empowerment through networking involves mutuality and reciprocity, personal support and sacrifice, caring and challenging, reunion and retribalization, and especially dedication among network members. These components were evident at HOT, MTP, and the Hispanic Family Counseling Program as we collaborated on providing our multicultural staff and trainees with peer support; opportunities for service coordination and community outreach; case conferences and training; and publication and presentation outlets.

As first director of the Latino Mental Health Service at Cambridge Hospital in 1983, my networking efforts focused on Latino/a urban health. In collaboration with an interagency network of health providers, including medical anthropologists, we worked to mutually support network members and to minimize the effects of stress and burnout associated with serving a generally disenfranchised and impoverished Latino/a community. We sought to address the general isolation of Latino/a health and human service workers and the lack of peer learning experiences in mainly non-Latino/a agencies. Among the characteristics of our network, the following were key: replacing competition with voluntary participation in interagency collaboration in a setting of limited resources; centralized case and service coordination from any one of several agency entry points and decentralized delivery; continuity of patient care insured by a service team who provided case follow-up as health providers turned over due to end of internship or residency, job changes, or geographic relocation; and the opportunity to openly ventilate and share the challenge in cross-cultural care (Carrillo & De La Cancela, 1992).

We are now at a historic juncture in which state health care reform proposals purport to provide expanded access to health services, the restoration of the physician's generalist functions, and greater emphasis on primary care. From a Latino/a perspective, the health service landscape has not moved too far from the conditions which gave rise to the network model in the late 1960s and early 1970s. We are still facing a traditional health services delivery system for visible ethnic racial groups which is costly, often maximizes social and cultural barriers, and minimizes access and availability.

Thus, it is not surprising that the health care proposals of the 1990s "reinvent" the concepts of community health, community oriented primary care and responsive medicine. For example, an urban medicine specialty has been promoted to train doctors to practice medicine for the underserved and correct the shortcomings of existing inner city health care systems (Nobbe, 1993). Even specialty oriented medical schools propose that faculty and graduates deliver health care services in inner city community-based outpatient clinics. From a financial perspective, entrepreneurs advise doctors to utilize a network approach to billing, purchasing, and the coordination of support personnel to realize significant economies of scale and make urban medical practice viable (Whigham-Desir, 1994). What is missing from the corporate health alliances and network models are the anthropological roots of "the network," i.e., the informal supports, the *compadrazgo/comadrazgo* (godparent-coparent) extended kin, input of consumers, community-based providers, and advocates engaged in participatory education and critical questioning embodied in earlier network models.

Health reform activism can benefit from the legacy and philosophy of the psychocultural network model developed at MTP and elsewhere. If primary care programs are to succeed, they must attend to prevention and behavioral change, school consultations and the epidemic addiction disorders that are plaguing our society, systems change and partnerships of cultural equity, and the quality of life for the poor, immigrants, and other medically underserved people of color. An empowerment network model can provide urban health policymakers, managers, and planners with opportunities to truly reform health care by doing more than taxing, cutting costs, and rationing health care through managed care and managed competition.

Network models should offer a principle-centered theory and practice that reject the quick-fix techniques that promise facile solutions to the complicated challenges of culturally competent health care for diverse populations. Many contemporary strategic organizational technologies such as total quality management and customer service orientations focus on techniques or vocabulary while largely ignoring people, content, purpose, and principles (Covey, 1990). Health care for all U.S. residents, including the undocumented, immigrant workers and disenfranchised citizens residing in Puerto Rico, the Virgin Islands, and the U.S. territories in the Pacific Islands should emanate from a public health vision that furthers the empowerment of all people (Freire, 1968). Real health empowerment for diverse communities requires both cooperative economies and community economic development.

The principle of wellness or *nuestro bienestar* has been proposed as a necessary paradigm shift in health service policy making for Latinos/as. *Nuestro bienestar* (literally translated "as our-well being") refers to a health care reform strategy based on collaboration and empowerment at the individual, family, and community level. It includes the use of natural networks for supporting comprehensive and integrated approaches to health maintenance. Networks such as schools and the workplace can provide health promotion programs (Carrillo, 1993).

Nuestro bienestar advocates funding for unified systems of care and multidisciplinary teams that respond to Latino/a definitions of mind and body, family and community, unity and continuity rather than administrative bureaucracies and organizations that create fragmented services by dividing people into their physical, social, emotional, and substance use problems. The *bienestar* approach advocates for capitated funding with clearly defined outcomes to replace categorical funding, and implies that comprehensive, culturally competent, biopsychosocial health delivery approaches will reduce the misuse of costly medical resources.

Latino/a health policy advocates from California, Texas, and New York call for family-based community health models that recognize women as significant health care managers, and children and adolescents as potential health promoters for their families and communities (Center for Health Policy Development [CHPD], 1993; Herrell, 1994). They encourage the use of other natural community networks and informal groups, along with community-based organizations which currently do not target health services, such as recreation centers, neighborhood sports teams, and public housing, as disease initiative sites.

SERVICE NETWORKS FOR THE COMMUNITY: AN AFRICAN AMERICAN EXAMPLE

Several years ago, the third author of this chapter was introduced to health networks in the Boston area as a psychology intern at the Minority Training Program in Clinical and Community Psychology (MTP). I sought admission to that internship to supplement a traditional learning experience that had not been meaningfully inclusive or affirmative of culturally and economically disenfranchised populations. From the outset, it was evident that networking, one of the cornerstones of the program, facilitated meaningful connections between African American students in psychology and senior level clinicians as well as viable connections to other psychology students and clinicians of color. This provided me and other trainees the culturally competent training and supervision lacking within standard/traditional programs in psychology.

Former interns and staff of the Minority Training Program have gone on to fill positions as community health administrators, clinicians, researchers, educators, and board members of various health and mental health resources throughout the United States and its territories in the Caribbean. Not only has this benefited the knowledge base and practical resource pool for the African American community, but also for other diverse communities as well.

The School Desegregation Response Project

A variety of field placements available for interns through the Minority Training Program facilitated the building and maintenance of viable networks because they were community based and addressed problems of prominent concern within the African American community. One of the placements where this was most evident was the School Desegregation Response Project (SDRP), a project responding to the school desegregation crisis in Boston occurring in the late 1970s. The SDRP was designed to train community mental health workers to intervene effectively in the school desegregation crisis. Training in crisis intervention was conducted at community health centers and other local social service centers with an emphasis on social, emotional, and environmental components of health. Those who completed the training were empowered to respond to parents, students, school personnel, police, and the larger community.

Via networking, the SDRP expanded to the cities of Cleveland and Los Angeles, where this model of collaboration, support, and crisis intervention was replicated in training mental health professionals and administrators. Thereafter, I conducted an evaluation of the training model, and found that the training model was effective, in preparing African American participants in particular, and within the community at large, in responding to crises, in facilitating the calming of fears and the appropriate channeling of anger and frustration, and in promoting ongoing planning and collaboration around school desegregation concerns.

Other Health Service Networks of Relevance for the African American Community

As a consultant on multiculturalism and diversity to two projects under the auspices of the Stone Center at Wellesley College, my networking efforts focused on promoting growth-fostering relationships guided by the relational theory of women's development (Miller, 1996). In conjunction with the Women in Prison Project (WIP), line staff and middle managers of a medium security facility were trained in the relational model in an effort to foster better working relationships with incarcerated women. All levels of the correctional staff and transitional community services (housing, counseling, health care, employment support, general follow-up) were consulted while developing the training model. This process was important in promoting valuable dialogue across levels which could potentially impact the incarcerated women. Focus groups for the women addressed issues leading to their incarceration, supported improved interpersonal relationships among them, and provided a forum for their concerns upon release. Improved relational skills and lower recidivism rates were the goals of the project. All of this had particular relevance for the African American women because of the connections they promoted. Even though they were the second largest ethnic group incarcerated at this facility, African American women tended to have and to expect the least support from their families (e.g., visits during incarceration and assurance of housing after release).

The Touchpoints Project focuses on educating new parents about infant and toddler development in conjunction with periodic well child visits. As consultant on diversity and multiculturalism to this project, I integrated principles of relational theory concerning women's development into the training of health practitioners in Brazelton's Touchpoint model (Brazelton, 1992). One of the training objectives was to foster positive relationships between parents from diverse backgrounds and to promote the use of preventive health services for children among health practitioners. A role of the consultant was to offer guidelines for developing relationships that pertained to ethnicity and culture. Health practitioners from several Boston area hospitals and health clinics participated in the pilot phase of this project. Many of the mothers they worked with were African American. This project expanded to health practitioners and administrators from other parts of the United States who were enabled in working with African American mothers. Since this project began in 1995, a longitudinal study of its effectiveness is not yet possible. However, nurse practitioners participating in the project have reported that the training has already made a difference in improving their relationships with mothers, and in increasing the rate of well child visits.

Other Potential Benefits of Health Service Networks for African Americans

Health service networks could also benefit the African American community by mobilizing residents to lobby against the advertising of cigarettes and alcohol in the community. Over the years, these substances have been glamorized to appeal to African American youth, thereby increasing addictions and compromising the health status of many in the community. In addition, health service networks could also play an advocacy role in seeking funding for research on the prevention and treatment of other illnesses that are prevalent in African American communities.

Some of what has already been described as the networking needs for Asian American and Latino/a communities also has relevance for African American communities. In view of the high prevalence in this community of hypertension, stroke, diabetes, breast cancer, homelessness, AIDS, substance abuse, and violence among young African American men, physical and social health indicators for this community need to be consulted. From an economic perspective, how realistic are standard benefits packages for the needs of those affected by these conditions? For example, is coverage adequate for low-income clients, and those with chronic or more serious conditions? How adequate is coverage for the black elderly or other low-income groups who may suffer from conditions that may require extended rehabilitative or nursing care? Some African Americans find their options for choosing an African American mental health provider limited under managed care plans. This is both in terms of availability for more common concerns and specialties (e.g., services to adolescents, the elderly, couples). As a consequence, a few pay out of pocket for mental health care, others prematurely terminate, and still others never receive the services they need. Details of how the financial terms of managed care plans operate for psychological care are unclear to some subscribers prior to helpseeking. After clarification, some subscribers become discouraged about the amount of copayment required and a limit on the number of approved psychotherapy sessions. Sometimes this results in not pursuing treatment at all. African Americans who live in suburban or rural communities often have to drive a considerable distance to receive culturally competent care. Furthermore, those who require specialized care and prefer to work with an African American provider may have to drive even further, which cancels out any likelihood of following through with care. Health networking can potentially influence managed care plans in identifying and including African American providers or ones with expertise in treating this population. Toward this end, more courses must be offered in conjunction with continuing education programs that address the psychological needs of African Americans.

The principles guiding and developing criteria for evaluating health plans must be ethnospecific to effectively respond to the needs of diverse populations. These examples emphasize the provider and consumer perspectives of how networks can be beneficial. Networks are consistent with the collective orientation within African American communities. In addition to the policy and systems emphasis in the other examples, the emphasis of this example is on how networks can enhance access to information and education, serve a supportive function, establish connections among resources, and facilitate collaboration among practitioners and consumers to confront institutional barriers to care.

CONCLUSION

In conclusion, the sociopolitical context provides a forum for examining the factors critical to reducing sociocultural barriers to health care. As the landscape of the macro system of health care changes, we need to ensure that we do not create new barriers or perpetuate old ones in the interest of change. Buzzwords such as "multicultural" and "cultural sensitivity" often just give lip service to the criteria of cultural competence.

From a macro level, we must advocate to promote change. We need to influence public policy to improve our systems of health care to ensure that they meet the needs of diverse communities and that communities are empowered in accessing competent health care. We must work as advocates from without, or as policymakers and administrators from within. While differences of culture and perspective remain and should be upheld, common themes provide the bond for communities of color to develop relevant solutions for reform.

Clearly, the policies suggested by activists must adhere to the spirit, commitment, survival, and maintenance of core cultural values indigenous to communities of color. It is this commitment that health care professionals ought to emulate in holding legislators, reformers, and policymakers accountable for delivering expanded access and coverage for the poor and medically underserved. The billions that the United States will spend to improve health care should be invested in culturally appropriate provider networks rather than powerful competitive private insurer networks.

Community health centers and public hospitals that have served as safety nets for poor, underserved, and "culturally different" patients, workers, and communities also must be guaranteed equitable funding in new health care economic policies. This is important because in many inner cities the public health centers and hospitals are major employers of people of color that contribute to the general economy of the community by providing jobs as well as serving their health needs.

Appropriate multilingual-multicultural social marketing of health promotion and disease prevention messages, higher level capitation payments, and penalties for delivering poor quality services or discriminating against people of color, the poor, and other disenfranchised groups must be enacted if we are to avoid the side effects of ill-conceived health reform policies.

By building on linkages among ethnocultural groups, their sense of community, social supports, and networks, community health networks can be empowering insofar as they expand the individual's or community's options to receive culturally competent service and enfranchise people by educating them as to their civil rights. Pitfalls include raising expectations that are met with inflexible institutional policies, or unexpected conflict that occurs between groups struggling over limited resources. The liabilities in following these recommendations are that we will be identified as irritants; the risk in not following them is that we will cease to be contributors to the preservation and growth of all people.

COMMENTARY

Ford H. Kuramoto

This chapter delineates community-oriented health service delivery and the inadequacy of existing health care delivery systems serving the United States' diverse populations. Most importantly, the chapter outlines recommendations for bringing about systemic social changes that would improve health care for all U.S. citizens.

Beginning with a historical perspective, the authors review the federally funded community health center and community mental health center movements which began in the mid-1960s. These two federally funded U.S. Department of Health and Human Services (then HEW) programs were part of the legacy of the Lyndon B. Johnson "Great Society" policies and the "War on Poverty." At that time, health and mental health service programs introduced a community-based system of care concept that included consumers in the governance structure. Federally funded community mental health centers stopped receiving funding in the mid-1970s when the Reagan administration ended the program with a mental health block grant. Related legislation and administrative regulations make it difficult for many projects serving people of color and other low-income populations to obtain funding and other resources.

The authors provide examples of barriers to effective implementation of community health centers using a series of contrasting pairs called dyadic perspectives. They illustrate the inconsistencies and tensions at various levels of a culturally competent system of care. Current health reform policy and practice, including health care financing, integrated service networks, and related policies fail to meet the health needs of a diverse U.S. population in a truly effective manner. Other factors include political forces such as immigration, welfare reform, and anti-affirmative action legislation.

The rapidly increasing cost of health care in the United States fermented the forces of change which made health care reform a presidential campaign issue in President Clinton's first term. The Clinton administration's far reaching, but politically overambitious proposal was ultimately rejected. This resulted in legislation focused solely on cost containment. Global economies and international business competition resulted in the downsizing of many segments of U.S. industry. The community health psychology perspective addresses the rising tide of retrograde, often racially motivated, and profit based efforts to reduce public entitlement and benefits. These reductions in government spending are made primarily at the cost of the poor who are disproportionately people of color. Welfare reform, immi-

gration reform, and anti-affirmative action legislation are aimed at reducing the number of people of color who are eligible for public benefits and services, while restricting those benefits to make the remaining services even less accessible and culturally competent. These policies were introduced by the "Contract with America" and leaders such as Newt Gingrich, Speaker of the House of Representatives. The question is where do these values and policies lead the United States as we enter the twenty-first century.

Health reform became an issue because both the public and private sectors believed that health care was too expensive, particularly with the increasing proportion of older persons covered by Medicare, Medicaid, and Social Security. Federal deficit reduction policies are reducing expenditures at the local, state, and national levels, thus providing declining health resources and other essential services. The huge proportion of the U.S. workforce being employed, but without any health insurance benefits was another factor. Adequate health care became such a large issue that policymakers and the public were desperate for some solution. The solution became managed care: cost containment. The managed care industry currently claims that it gave policymakers and the public what they asked for: reduced health costs.

However, the controversy continues because many health care consumers in both the private and public sectors are very dissatisfied with the quality and extent of care. Disillusionment is spreading. Consumers have less access to quality care, providers are forced into provider groups with limited flexibility regarding clinical decisions, and the marketplace has created a chaotic series of mergers and changes in providers. Cost containment has also threatened the safety net of community-based health and social service providers that are essential resources for people of color and other low-income populations.

Moreover, cost containment has brought a re-emphasis on the medical model approach with the narrowing focus based on "medical necessity." Nontraditional, holistic services that are useful for multicultural populations are even more limited and difficult to obtain. The whole mental health and substance abuse prevention and treatment areas of care are even more limited in both public and private sectors. Consumers of health, mental health, and substance abuse services in both the public and private sectors are understandably confused about their options and increasingly dissatisfied with their declining access to services. Prevention is virtually eliminated from most cost containment systems where the emphasis is on reducing expenditures for medical treatment.

Finally, these policies raise basic questions regarding values and priorities—what does the United States stand for? In essence, the issues are: who "belongs" and will all U.S. residents be equal? The U.S. response to these issues defines what we as a society currently stand for, the culture of the nation, and whether the changing political and policy landscape has brought us to a better place.

The authors offer solutions to health care reform. They provide examples and recommendations for optimum health and well-being through community oriented health care. A community health psychology perspective can promote health at individual, family, group, and community levels. Reducing sociocultural barriers to health care at the micro and macro levels is a very complex challenge. Advocacy at many levels will be required in order to create the systemic changes needed to overcome the many sociocultural barriers to health and well-being.

Health reform discussion from a total systems approach is a particularly important, timely, illuminating contribution to this topic of national debate. The authors' specific ethnic group discussions regarding the current application of health reform policies is an extremely valuable contribution to the literature. Their community health psychology perspective will help strengthen our society through building stronger, healthier, more productive communities that will help the United States in the twenty-first century. The caveat is that for the community health psychology perspective to be truly effective, the psychology field must reinvent itself and fully embrace this perspective in order to lead other providers, consumers, and policymakers in this crucial social movement.

5

Culturally Competent Community Health Psychology: A Systemic Approach

Yvonne M. Jenkins,
Victor De La Cancela, and Jean Lau Chin

Community health psychology moves beyond a focus on single factors that influence the individual status of the client to larger systems that influence the incidence of illness, availability of services, and quality of care for entire communities. In addition, this timely and innovative primary care specialty is concerned with the reform of health systems to promote the overall well-being of communities. We believe that culture is central to the practice of community health psychology because it may be used to guide service delivery and health reform. We also believe that the diversity in communities must be acknowledged and effectively responded to through policy and systemic perspectives in health psychology. Therefore, with culturally competent practice as its guiding principle, this chapter discusses culturally competent community health psychology. Furthermore, it addresses a need to diversify the psychologist health services provider's role to achieve this. Additionally, attention is paid to policy, priorities, and regulatory issues that acknowledge diversity and facilitate culturally competent approaches to care. We believe that diversification of the psychologist's role and acknowledgment of diversity promotes the overall health and well-being of underserved communities.

CULTURALLY COMPETENT
COMMUNITY HEALTH PSYCHOLOGY

Culturally competent community health psychology involves an integration of natural support systems and indigenous provider networks into health and public health practice, community outreach and advocacy, and holistic/biopsychosocial approaches that attend to ethnomedical and alternative medical systems. Also, the service delivery, organization, and administration of culturally competent practice is informed by comparative health care analysis and the communities served. To achieve this end, any number of nonstandard processes and mechanisms that incorporate the aforementioned approaches may be considered. These may include the use of paraprofessional providers, regular use of schools, churches, community centers, and community health fairs and forums as outreach and liaison mechanisms, enlisting the support of community leaders, politicians, and health administrators for advocacy purposes, and approaches that incorporate ethnomedical and alternative medical systems such as acupuncture, meditation, and naturopathy. Along with focus groups and other nonmainstream resources, these processes and mechanisms also serve to inform culturally competent service delivery, organization, and administration.

More often than not, our systems do not take into consideration the needs of non-English–speaking populations. Furthermore, what is believed to be culturally competent care for these populations is usually reduced to the provision of interpretation services alone. Consequently, members of diverse cultures with adequate English skills generally utilize health care systems with little expectation that there will be an understanding of culture. Moreover, many English-speaking members of diverse groups teach themselves to be culture-neutral while utilizing the health care system. Yet, this defies the knowledge that cultural beliefs, values, and practices contribute to health beliefs, values, and practices.

Many current health policies, regulatory issues, and health care priorities neglect the needs of much of the middle-class and the most oppressed groups in society. These are often out of synchrony with the needs of diverse communities and impede the development of systematic perspectives, culturally competent approaches, and favorable outcomes to care.

RATIONALE FOR THE ROLE DIVERSIFICATION OF PSYCHOLOGIST HEALTH SERVICE PROVIDERS

Diverse communities tend to be found in inner city areas that are primarily populated by the poor, working class, and women. The composition of these areas is largely a consequence of poverty or modest socioeconomic status, vulnerability to longstanding societal problems (e.g., racism, prejudice, discrimination), and internalization of oppression. Of particular relevance to our focus is the unfortunate reality that these groups are commonly shortchanged by health care systems constructed on frameworks that, from a cultural perspective, conflict with their lived experiences. Consequently, residents of these areas are likely to encounter: inadequate health care (medical and psychological), inadequate insurance plans; unaffordable and untimely health care; frequent visits to medical practitioners; too few sessions with private psychological practitioners; an inability to access private treatment; and radical or invasive medical procedures as opposed to preventative measures, particularly if chronically or seriously ill (Smith & Burns, 1993).

There are instances where adaptive ethnocultural mechanisms (e.g., indigenous support systems, the extended family) compensate for these barriers. However, there are far too many instances where the neglect of early signs of dysfunction or illness leads to the development of more serious and chronic health and psychological problems, chemical dependency, violence, or other debilitating conditions. Not only does role diversification for psychologist health services providers create opportunities within the field but it also makes the value of the profession evident to others outside the field. Community health psychologists have the potential to play a central role in eradicating the neglect that is so commonly suffered by diverse communities. To achieve this, however, the role of the health psychologist must expand beyond that of therapist or counselor. One area in which the field of psychology is expanding is nonclinically oriented consultation.

Expanding the Role of Consultant

Even though acceptance of the utility of psychologists has varied among public health practitioners, members of this profession have been effectively used as consultants on a variety of public health problems despite the numerous practical challenges they have encountered (Matthews & Ridgeway, 1984). According to Leviton (Leviton, 1995), opportunities for integrating psychology with public health are created by the focus on incremental improvements via state-stage modeling. These opportunities focus on whether existing frameworks or models are integrated logically and consistently, and the efficacy of public health systems. The expertise of psychologists is used for improving existing service delivery systems, programs, and policies. The expertise of psychologists has also been used for developing techniques that improve adherence to treatment for hypertension (Weinstein & Stason, 1976). Furthermore, psychologists have aided with adapting the analysis of transitional probabilities for the practice of public health in a variety of areas. These have ranged from immunization to exercise (Russell, 1985) to needle exchange programs (Kaplan & Brandeau, 1994) to rodent control (Leviton, Chen, Marsh, & Talbott, 1993). In addition, psychologists have enhanced communication about health and safety problems (Lefebvre & Flora, 1988). In this era where the focus on wellness is more prominent than ever before, clearly there are also opportunities for psychologists to shape messages for lifestyle change and relevant consequences that are of importance to policymakers. For example, there are opportunities to translate the efficacy of behavioral interventions into practical implications that influence more cost-effective services. Finally, Leviton (Leviton, 1995) emphasizes that psychologists have opportunities to impact entire communities through social marketing, the marshaling of varied sources of community support, and collaboration with medical professionals and professionals in the field of public health.

Opportunities for Exploration

Other opportunities exist for psychologists to participate in health and mental health services. These include organization and management, psychoeducation and training, planning and policy development, activism, research, and publishing. With these opportunities in mind, this chapter discusses policy, regulatory issues, and priorities that currently preclude the development of systematic perspectives and approaches that facilitate culturally competent psychological health care systems. It is our intent that this focus may serve as a catalyst for new and progressive ideas on the role of health psychologists in the future, and that health psychologists will become more proactive and diversified in responding to the needs of diverse communities.

POLICY, REGULATORY ISSUES, AND
HEALTH CARE PRIORITIES

In view of the shift of public and private health care systems to managed care and the impact of this shift on the delivery of psychological and public health services, prevention, and cost effectiveness are now more critical than ever before. These tasks cannot be achieved in the absence of culturally competent care. An absence of culturally competent care is associated with an increased incidence of illness and the need for more expensive health procedures and interventions. Community input on such issues as the needs of a particular community and culture-specific health practices, culturally relevant research data, and culturally competent administrative agencies and providers are needed to influence policy that promotes culturally competent care. Evidence of such care will initially be apparent in high utilization rates for preventive health care and a decline in acute health care costs over time. Clearly, psychologists as health service providers do much to promote health maintenance, the treatment of serious health problems, and the reduction of health care costs. For these reasons, it is advantageous for health policy to include provisions for insuring the availability of psychologists and their services to diverse populations. As such, culturally competent psychological care can be facilitated by such policy modifications as the following:

1. Increased integration of psychological services with health care to facilitate prevention and lower health care costs. When provided in a timely manner, the provision of psychological services has the potential to prevent significant psychological deterioration and the development of significant adjustment, medical, and safety problems. There is considerable evidence that psychologists have contributed to a dramatic reduction in health costs for alcoholics and recovering surgery patients (Matthews & Ridgeway, 1984; Suinn, 1996; Wells, Howard, Nowlin, & Vargas, 1986). Suinn (Suinn, 1996) emphasizes that psychologists have developed major behavioral medicine intervention programs that target cessation of smoking, excessive drinking, overeating, and failure to use seat belts, while other programs promote hypertension control and low impact exercise. Furthermore, psychologists are making significant contributions to the areas of pain management and the treatment of cardiovascular disease, diabetes, cancer, arthritis, and HIV infection and AIDS. In the near future, psychologists are expected to make similar contributions to prevention involving the immune system.

One particularly innovative example of the application of culturally competent behavioral intervention by psychologists and other mental health professionals is in the treatment of hypertension. A support group for African American graduate students and employees at an Ivy League university meets on a weekly basis to support adherence to medical, psychological, and lifestyle interventions that lower risks inherent to hypertension. This fine example of culturally competent practice responds to the particularly high incidence of hypertension among African Americans. The group integrates biofeedback, relaxation training, consistent attention to diet and exercise, blood pressure monitoring, and attention to social problems associated with racial status and related social problems that influence elevated stress levels for African Americans.

2. More expansive coverage for mental health and chemical dependency services. Although health insurance is a strong predictor of whether one seeks mental health care, this benefit is not covered by many health insurance policies (Glied & Kofman, 1995). Mental health coverage is far more limited than that for medical or surgical services. Stricter limits are set on outpatient mental health visits and hospital days along with higher copayments and higher cost sharing in order to limit costs to insurers (Sharfstein, Stoline, & Goldman, 1993). This impacts on diverse communities disproportionately since poverty tends to be higher in these areas and economic resources more limited than what is typically available in suburban communities. Some employment-based insurance plans offer up to 90 visits a year with a 50% copayment (Boyle & Callahan, 1993). Plans at the upper limit of this continuum are clearly the exception. However, most are not as generous and limit the outpatient benefit to $500 per calendar year, which covers an average of 6 to 10 visits. This is sufficient for crisis intervention or transient conditions manifested by basically healthy individuals that are amenable to brief treatment. Yet, such limited coverage is grossly inadequate for sustaining care for those with more serious and chronic problems.

Outpatient mental health packages offered by health maintenance organizations (HMOs) are restricted to 20 to 30 visits per calendar year with a 50% copayment. However, these are the most generous exceptions in that far more are restricted to six sessions or fewer. Thereafter, providers are usually required to periodically submit time consuming paperwork for gatekeeper analysis and utilization review that assess the need for continued care. This process seems to overlook the reality that "general health care . . . exists within the primary domain of psychology" (Suinn, 1996). There are times when the gatekeeper-utilization review process strains the therapeutic relationship by disrupting the treatment process and causing undue anxiety to the recipient of care. Often the therapist is put in an ethical bind while awaiting authorization for continuation. Some rejected requests for the authorization of continuing care result in premature termination since even sliding fee requirements are more than some clients can afford to pay out of pocket. Also, to protect the confidentiality of the client and to avoid insurance and HMO restrictions on preexisting conditions, psychologists, and other mental health providers are hesitant to indicate full diagnoses on requests for services and claim forms. Medicaid is restrictive in that its low fees often prevent those in the most distress from receiving care from private practitioners on the extended basis typically necessary for favorable outcomes. Even more restricted are those persons with no insurance coverage. This population is 40% as likely as Medicaid recipients to seek mental health care (Horgan, 1985). While Medicare pays higher fees than Medicaid, this resource is targeted for the elderly, a population that is often beset by chronic and serious health problems. Even so, Medicare requires copayments and does not cover the cost of medications. Furthermore, stricter limits are set on outpatient visits and hospital days along with higher copayments and cost sharing (Sharfstein et al., 1993).

For those plagued by a combination of personal and societal problems, there is only enough coverage for "putting out fires" until the next crisis occurs. Yet, at a more significant level, such limited coverage leaves little, if any, opportunity for meaningful exploration or sustained behavioral change. Moreover, it is unlikely to enable recipients of care to become social change agents given the necessity to work towards resolution of societal problems on both individual and collective levels. For example, some insurance companies have adopted a particularly unfair stance toward women in the denial of health benefits where there is pre-existing evidence of partner/spousal abuse. When there is evidence of such abuse, timely contacts with health care providers have possibilities for leading to contacts with vital social services (e.g., shelters, support groups, job counseling, and placement) that could facilitate safety and autonomy. Also, for obvious reasons, the availability of these supportive services is in the best interest of children and adolescents. Clearly, current limits on mental health coverage have risky implications when cost effectiveness is preferred over the psychological and physical well-being of individuals, families, and communities.

3. Equalize status between mental health and medical benefits. Reform of health coverage must involve advancing mental health benefits to a more equitable status with medical coverage. This

would involve higher cost sharing for psychotherapy and pharmacotherapy and the inclusion of subsidies to eliminate the burden of cost sharing for the poor. Furthermore, in view of the value of early intervention, unlimited coverage needs to be available to children and adolescents. In addition, comprehensive psychological coverage is essential for those with pre-existing conditions.

Other Policy Issues for Various Levels of Intervention

Several policy issues that impact persons with psychological and chemical dependency disorders as well as health services providers have been identified by De La Cancela (Eisenberg, 1992) elsewhere. Those of the first group include: their "vulnerable population" status and the stigma associated with their illnesses which have prevented meaningful consumer participation in the design of managed care programs; the definitions of community prevention and clinical preventive services on federal and state levels and how these differ from specialized views of private health care management companies; how the use of savings from a capitation system can pay for nontraditional prevention services (e.g., peer support groups, counseling for children who are at risk due to their parents' socioeconomic status); the use of experienced, community-based providers with a positive track record in addressing special needs of at risk or culturally diverse populations; and how managed care systems must promote current access to preventive mental health and chemical dependency care to control costs in the future.

Policy issues for health services providers in the aforementioned areas include: appropriate reimbursement rates for clinical preventive services and payment for support services; access to specialized prevention information and technical support to expand prevention expertise; and expansion of nontraditional services.

Progressive changes for public health and state systems and proposed strategies for implementing these through policy are necessary. At the public health level, policy is needed to define and ensure the promotion of mental health, substance abuse, and disease prevention services. Among those strategies suggested for implementation are: data collection and analysis, assessment of the expertise and experience of providers and preventionists, training providers in prevention, and recruitment of culturally competent providers. At the state level, bureaucratic obstacles, barriers, "turfing," threats, and other forms of institutional resistance to change need to be overcome by state mental health, chemical dependency, and Medicaid agencies. Information regarding innovative collaboration models should be shared between and within states to impact prevention and managed care integration and the design of a basic prevention care benefits package that would be delineated in contracts developed with private managed care companies. Public health, mental health, and substance abuse providers also must be assisted with developing new aspects of practice (i.e., preventive care, cultural competence, consumer partnership, effective business management) and a more progressive perspective of what constitutes ethical practice.

Active Attention to Preventive Health Care Services for Women of Color

Cervical cancer, breast cancer, high blood pressure, and illnesses associated with smoking (disease, lung cancer) are the main causes of death for women. Screening tests (e.g., pap test, mammogram, blood pressure check) and regular physical examinations have the potential to lower the morbidity and mortality associated with these conditions. Yet, utilization of screening tests and annual physical exams is much lower for women of color than for Caucasian women. This is associated with the lack of insurance benefits and the lack of a usual source of health care.

The Commonwealth Fund Commission (Glied & Koffman, 1995) reports finding that women of color were less likely than Caucasian women to be screened for breast cancer with Asian women as the least likely group (55%). Latinas have the second largest group of women who had not been screened (43%), with 37% of African American women reporting never being screened for cervical cancer.

Women of color constitute a large percentage of the poor. Women with few economic resources are less likely to be screened than women with higher incomes. This is particularly evident with screening for breast cancer. For example, 64% of women below the poverty level had not had a mammogram in two years.

In view of the high incidence of hypertension in African American communities, it is particularly encouraging that 82% of African American women aged 18 and older were screened for this illness. This was followed by 80% of Caucasian women, 74% of Latinas, and 73% of Asian women. These utilization patterns for women of color have the following policy implications:

- clinical outreach and education programs need to include community input on how to make such programs both culturally syntonic and targeted to this population; similar age-appropriate programs should be designed for girls that continue throughout adolescence to promote attention to healthy self-caretaking behavior earlier in life;

- full health insurance for recommended levels of preventive service would reduce barriers that block women from being screened;
- active and timely follow-up for both recent and missed appointments need to be systematized to maintain the interpersonal and clinical connection that promotes the health and well-being of this population.

Active Attention to Preventive Health Care Services for Men of Color

In view of the medical and psychosocial issues for men (and boys) of color that have been mentioned previously, it is obvious that this population could also benefit from policy that is similar to that proposed for women (and girls) of color above. Screening for prostate cancer, HIV infection and AIDS, hypertension, heart disease, diabetes, and overall stress level would be particularly useful to this population. In addition, since men are reportedly less likely than women to seek preventive health care, policy that supports the design of outreach and education programs focused specifically on men's health in a manner that appeals to men of color is essential. Obviously the input of this population would be critical for shaping such policy, in designing effective programs, and to promote self-esteem development within this population.

A Sound Research Data Base

In order to facilitate prevention and cost-effective care in diverse communities, a relevant, valid, and reliable research database is needed to guide the determination of priorities, policymaking, and service delivery. The design of such projects must be in the best interests of the communities served as opposed to the economic interests of universities, hospitals, or other institutions that house such projects. The input of the communities served and culturally competent health psychologists is essential to achieving outcomes that have practical and progressive value for diverse communities. Therefore, periodic attention to the following issues could be instructive: What sociopsychological impact does managed care have on the health and well-being of people of color? Is managed care, as currently practiced, truly cost effective (i.e., in relation to hospitalization costs subsequent to short term care)? What input do subscribers have on ways to improve this benefit? What factors (cultural, social, contextual) influence illness and health (sociopsychological and physical)? What service utilization patterns exist for what specific groups? Which groups tend to use psychological services? Which groups need services but tend not to use them? What alternatives to standard/mainstream services (mental health, medical) are used by which groups? What are the implications for outreach, health education, and psychoeducation services? How do choices of services differ by racial/ethnic/cultural group, gender, age, diagnosis, location, and socioeconomic status? What factors influence these choices? Which types of services have not been delivered in the best interest of diverse populations? What are some effective applied psychology strategies for enabling practitioners and mental health facilities to make effective transitions to managed care?

In the public sector it would be useful to explore whether health reform impacts men and women differentially. It would also be useful to explore how the "carving out" of benefits impacts the coordination of mental health care across providers. What are the implications of integrated versus carved out behavioral health benefits for community health psychology? Are there ways in which psychological services, natural support systems, and public and private institutions (e.g., police departments, after school programs, social services, churches, local businesses, universities) can work together effectively in the delivery of psychological health services?

Finally, in both public and private sectors it would be useful to explore how contextual factors (e.g., culture, race, ethnicity, poverty) influence psychosocial and physical health. Exploration of the following issues could benefit system-wide reform: What subgroups (e.g., children, the elderly) within which particular ethnocultural groups tend to be without health care coverage? What percentage of the population of diverse communities is limited by coverage with pre-existing clauses? Is coverage available for those who have recently experienced a crisis? How do cultural, societal, and informational factors impact on the use of care? What social supports (e.g., child care, transportation, home visits, flexible appointments, subsidized phone services) would facilitate access to care for what specific populations (e.g., the elderly, women)? How consistent is the demographic makeup of providers with that of the community served? What supportive services are available to high-risk groups (e.g., victims of abuse, children of substance abusers, family caregivers of seriously ill persons, close relatives of those with major mental illnesses)? What are the most effective ways to eradicate the stigma and shame associated with help seeking? What are the most effective ways to reach out to groups who have not tended to seek preventive and clinical services (e.g., men of color, pregnant teens, those groups which have tended to forego screening for HIV infection and AIDS).

Glied and Kofman's (Glied & Kofman, 1995) discussion of risks that proposals for mental health reform pose for women have applicability to developing culturally competent research on health coverage for diverse communities. They contend that "[a] careful assessment of alternative sources of psychosocial care . . . [for those unable to] afford [direct payment] should precede any wholesale shift in coverage" (p. 92). What is needed, they suggest, is an analysis of the effect of gatekeepers on the use of mental health services with results presented by gender, ethnicity, and diagnosis. This would be helpful for determining whether less assertive recipients of care, who internalize their conditions, may give up rather than struggle with bureaucratic procedures.

Explore Policy Implications of Illness

From a public health perspective, it would be worthwhile to explore the policy implications of illness for specific communities. For example, what policy needs are suggested by data for domestic violence, sexually transmitted diseases, or substance abuse among pregnant mothers? A culturally competent approach to addressing these issues would be guided by knowledge of the world view, cultural values, and health-related needs of the community, accurate and relevant research data, and effective integration of psychological, medical, and social services.

Community Input on the Definition of Needs

What has at times resulted in a mismatch between needs and services may be linked to policymakers' and practitioners' lack of authentic familiarity with the communities serviced. By avoiding the input of residents, those in power have often inaccurately perceived the needs and lifestyles (inclusive of ethnocultural influences) of inner-city communities. Models of care that are consistent with the needs and values of the dominant cultural group have usually been indiscriminately applied to all groups regardless of any diversity that might have existed between the dominant group and pluralistic populations. In view of these very important differences and inflexible approaches to care, clearly the fit between needs and services has been poor.

The attempt to respond to needs without the input of the community and adherence to culturally dystonic approaches to care can be quite costly. One fairly common example of this is evident in some of the publicly funded nutrition programs. For example, the WIC Program offers milk, cheese, and other commodities to its recipients. Yet, since cheese is not among the dietary preferences for Chinese communities, it is rarely used. Even so, this practice continues. Instead it would be more reasonable to explore what other commodity would be more suitable for use in Chinese communities to achieve similar nutrition outcomes. Another example of overlooking the importance of community input to intervention is apparent in the assumption that homes for the aged are *always* preferable to other options for residential care. This assumption is contrary to the strong family orientations of African Americans, Latinos/as, and Asians. Elder day care in one's own community, a less costly option, is a more culturally syntonic option for these groups when no relative is available to take care of a loved one. It is also important to recognize that the Western notion of prevention is difficult for some diverse populations to embrace. For example, after several months of meeting with a therapist on an intermittent basis, a United States citizen from India expressed discomfort with developing a treatment contract that included psychotherapy sessions for times other than crises. This was in response to her therapist's efforts to explore her reticence about scheduling sessions for more often than once a month. The woman explained that she had come from a background of poverty which made her feel that more frequent sessions would be too indulgent and a careless use of a health resource. Even though she acknowledged that she had far more resources at present than she did while growing up in India, it was obvious that her childhood and adolescence there still had an impact on this aspect of her world view. With this in mind, a treatment contract oriented toward prevention and support was developed that was more consistent with her comfort level.

These examples suggest that health care choices guided by culture-specific input enhance the relationship between caregiver and consumer, as well as the psychological and physical well-being of the consumer. In addition, such input promotes the continuity of care that facilitates prevention and is therefore more cost-effective than culturally dystonic models of care. For these reasons, the input of consumers is essential to the development of policy for service delivery. Culturally competent care calls for Western notions of prevention and acceptable health services practices to be redefined in ways that truly empower diverse communities through embracing diversity.

Community input might also make more evident the need for more collaboration between psychologists and medical practitioners. For example, it has been repeatedly demonstrated that pluralistic populations are more likely to initiate contact with medical practitioners than psychologists. Furthermore, since shame and stigma continue to be associated with psychological problems, some suffer in silence or without ever reaching out for help. Yet, medical practitioners often lack the skills to diagnose psychological problems (Eisenberg, 1992; Mechanic, 1990). Furthermore, some practitioners lack the sensitivity and social competence "to identify with, empathize with, and take interest in psychosocial aspects of health" (Wallis, 1992). In addition, differential needs and utilization patterns often tend to be overlooked. Too often these inadequacies result in missed opportunities for intervention that make the difference between achieving psychological and physical health and gradual deterioration. It seems that systematic collaboration between psychologists and health practitioners is both an ethical and practical necessity. With the input of the community and culturally competent health psychologists, a congruent match between needs and services does, indeed, seem possible. Obviously, the potential for such input to prevent the incidence of serious illness (i.e., physical and psychosocial) could benefit consumers as well as insurers.

Emphasis on Care at Every Stage of the Life Cycle

As stated in Chapter Two, the traditional medical care structure places emphasis on the provision of care at the beginning and final stages of the life cycle. Even so, certain segments of the population, during these and interim stages of the life cycle, receive little if any timely health care and find comprehensive health care virtually inaccessible. Among those populations that are routinely underserved are the poor, uneducated and mentally retarded, pregnant adolescents and their partners, immigrants, men of color, migrant workers, and residents of rural areas. It would be wise to actively elicit the input of these groups or advocates to influence early case finding, timely intervention, and follow-up care.

PRIORITIES FOR DIVERSE COMMUNITIES

Priorities for diverse communities must be oriented toward making medical and psychological health care more accessible, culturally competent, and affordable. Service delivery must be guided by the needs of residents as well as significant ethnocultural and social considerations. Therefore, ethnocultural world views, values, social class, folk healing modalities, and the intergenerational relationship of specific groups with traditional medicine and standard psychological care in the United States must be considered.

In view of these considerations, the first priority is to examine the relevance and effectiveness of health-related programs and services in both the public and private sectors. The expertise of psychologists is central to achieving this objective. To make medical and psychological care more accessible and culturally relevant at the state level would involve evaluating and developing new policies associated with medical, psychological, and social health care in managed care systems when appropriate. It would also involve evaluating individual, organizational, and community benefits of preventive health and psychological health care, and determining what specific preventive services have worked most effectively in specific service delivery settings. In addition to achieving the aforementioned tasks, psychologists could also play vital roles in research design, data collection and analysis, and, where appropriate, recruiting and training other professionals, folk providers, and preventionists as community health psychology associates.

Secondly, the policy, regulatory issues, and health care priorities highlighted earlier in this chapter suggest that broad health and social services policy issues affecting consumers of care must be considered by those at every level of the health care system. Psychologists could be instrumental in implementing more meaningful consumer participation in the design of managed care programs and health insurance programs. Consumer participation is particularly needed in the redefinition of *prevention* at community, clinical, and federal/state levels. It is also important to determine how this may differ from specialized views of private health care management and how these differences, views, and philosophical underpinnings can be acknowledged, negotiated, and reframed toward partnering for culturally competent, cost-effective health services.

Some related regulatory issues to be addressed include: the formulation of a plan for using savings from a capitation system to pay for nontraditional prevention services; the development of directories that include experienced community-based providers organized by areas of expertise, interests, and discipline; and a plan for how managed care systems can promote better access to preventive mental health and substance abuse care.

A third priority is to support the professional development and well-being of health services providers. Policy must be developed to offer appropriate reimbursement rates to providers for clinical and supportive services designed to promote prevention. In addition, steps must be taken to increase access to specialized physical, psychological, social health, and folk/nontraditional medicine information and technical support oriented to prevention. Steps must also be taken to expand nontraditional services and to develop appropriate reimbursement rates for these. Furthermore, in view of the fact that underserved populations often lack access to health care coverage, more affordable fee-for-service opportunities need to be offered. Not only would this make care available to those who might not otherwise receive it but it would create more opportunities for health services providers. Lastly, stipends for continuing education relevant to prevention, diversity, and self-care (e.g., decreasing burnout) must be made available.

From a public health perspective, an important regulatory mechanism would involve managing the delivery of the best quality of preventive psychological, medical, and social health care. At the community health level, attention to local and prevailing standards of service delivery, consumer empowerment, and satisfaction is necessary. More attention to the development of social health programs (e.g., violence prevention, anger management, diversity acknowledgment) is needed in particular.

At the state level, a priority for all levels of care is to overcome institutional resistance to change. To achieve this, psychologists may become involved in disseminating information regarding innovative collaboration models to impact future prevention and managed care integration developments. In addition, states must design a basic prevention care benefits package that can be delineated in contracts developed with private managed care companies. An ultimate challenge for states is to assist public health, medical, and psychological health providers to develop new definitions of practice including preventive care, cultural competence, consumer partnerships, and good business management skills.

Finally, to make mental health services more affordable to residents of inner city communities, insurers must make it a priority to advance psychological, behavioral medicine, and social health coverage to a status more equitable with medical coverage so that general and specialty psychological care can be appropriately available and accessible to those who need it. In addition, potential subscribers need to be protected from exclusionary clauses for pre-existing conditions as well as prior evidence of spousal/domestic partner abuse.

CONCLUSION

In conclusion, in order to serve diverse communities effectively health policy and practice systems must reflect the needs of those served so that it is respectful of unique ethnocultural influences. To achieve this, the strengths of both traditional and folk/ethnomedicine, and natural support systems must be integrated appropriately to provide culturally competent care. This also requires increased collaboration between psychologists and other health providers. The role diversification of psychologists expands opportunities for this profession to impact progressively relevant policy development, outreach, management and practice, and research.

COMMENTARY

Carlos Molina

The chapter presents the effectiveness of using culturally competent psychologists to deliver mental health services, and argues for expanding their functions to include health promotion and disease prevention efforts targeted at people of color. The authors recommend that culturally competent psychologists be included in all aspects of health care delivery systems and research. These are sound recommendations, and make perfectly good sense. However, psychologists skilled in multiculturalism are only part of the solution to reach out successfully to ethnic/racial populations. Equally important is increasing the pool of other culturally competent health professionals (health educators and medical care providers).

Public health data have repeatedly shown that applying behavioral medicine's strategies targeted at primary and secondary preventive health behaviors, as delineated by the authors, can save more lives and reduce health care and societal costs more dramatically than any new curative discovery by biomedical research. However, there exists a dearth of health promotion programs (smoking cessation, low-risk drinking, healthy eating, seat belt use, etc.) that target ethnic/racial populations. As a means of increasing culturally-specific health promotion programs, the authors correctly call for the inclusion of culturally competent health psychologists in the development, delivery, and evaluation of these programs.

It is through culture that people around the world communicate their illnesses and their well-being. A community's culture prescribes and influences the prevention and healing behaviors for its people. It stands to reason that working within the cultural paradigm of the population being served will only increase the probability of successful outcomes for public health strategies and medical care interventions. However, in order to increase the pool of culturally sensitive psychologists, and other health professionals, graduate programs, medical schools, and health professions schools need to infuse their curricula with appropriate language and cultural education.

The chapter recognizes that, in addition to cultural barriers, there are other barriers that prevent ethnic/racial populations from accessing mental health and other health services. Torrey's (1968) explanation of the underutilization of mental health services by Mexican Americans can be applied to other Latino/a groups and other ethnic/racial populations. It includes geographic inaccessibility, language barriers, the class-bound values of the therapist, and the culture-bound values of the therapist. My work with diverse populations (Molina & Aguirre-Molina, 1994) also suggests that it is applicable to all health services, and is in synchrony with this chapter's discussion of the cultural, linguistic, economic, and societal factors that influence access.

6

Community Health Psychology's Strategic Planning for Health Care Reform: The Empowerment Solution

Victor De La Cancela

With the enactment of numerous state Medicaid Managed Care initiatives* many public health and hospitals systems find themselves in the uncustomary position of having to compete for Medicaid patients with private hospitals who previously made little effort to serve such patients. Currently, these providers, collectively known as the "safety net"—public hospitals, community and migrant health centers, and others who provide health care for the poor and underserved urban and rural communities (NYCHHC, 1989) obtain a significant percentage of their patient base from Medicaid recipients; this Medicaid population accounts for the majority of their revenue. The problem for safety net public agencies/systems is how to retain a Medicaid base under state Medicaid reform or how to implement Medicaid Managed Care† in a new competitive environment.

This situation occurs as many agencies are attempting to become

---

*State Medicaid Managed Care is one of the states' most significant health care initiatives of the past decade, and aims to contain the growth rate of expenditures for Medicaid recipients through their enrollment in voluntary and mandatory managed care programs.

†Medicaid Managed Care is the health care system often established by state law/state agency regulation, to provide well coordinated primary care to *Medicaid* patients.

more fiscally autonomous from local government, are being restructured through downsizing and attrition, or experiencing budget reduction and other cost controls. Thus, the success of the safety net with respect to Medicaid Managed Care is a key to the future fiscal health of municipal/state health systems. Yet current re-inventing/re-engineering movements have created a lapse in leadership as it relates to the promotion, implementation, and oversight of Medicaid Managed Care education. Community health psychology can meet this challenge by establishing managed care education interventions to support safety net facilities in making the Medicaid Managed Care effort succeed. It is the intent of this manuscript to both provide a case study of the results of this process and to provide by illustration a conceptual framework for community health psychologists, educators, managers, and staff to understand and constructively handle the individual and organizational impact of "dramatic change" engendered by state mandated health care reform (Wilkenfeld, 1994).

Strategic planning for health care reform is significantly linked to community health psychology's overarching themes of empowerment for communities of color given the historic efforts of safety net providers in overcoming the reality of provider reluctance toward serving low-income populations of color, recent immigrants, undocumented persons, and the homeless because of the complicated, severe, and multifaceted nature of their health. These factors require that safety net providers be allocated adequate resources for the development of sufficient and culturally competent health education programs to help them reorient and educate the poor populations they serve to make healthy choices and decisions in engaging systems of managed care (Harden, 1993).

Toward this end, community health psychology can help to ensure that:

- safety net services are readily accessible and geared to meet the needs of diverse target audiences;
- the benefits of safety net managed care services are communicated effectively to those who can most benefit from the services;
- the mission of safety net leadership to help all facilities/network staff to develop a common vision of managed care* is continued, and;

---

*Managed care generally refers to organized health care delivery systems that coordinate use of services, directly/indirectly by referral, and case management through a single entry point into the system—the primary care practitioner.

- the commitment of all stakeholders to achieve maximum success in the continued growth of managed care.

Community health psychology can utilize a social marketing approach to help the safety net implement managed care and provide responsive service to present and potential customers and consumers of Medicaid Managed Care services. Social marketing is a research based process used to bring about the adoption or acceptability of ideas or practices. It involves a consumer orientation, voluntary exchanges of ideas or practices for a perceived benefit, audience analysis and segmentation, formative research, process tracking to assess utilization trends, and management (Green & Kreuter, 1991). Marketing activities include the education of safety net staff to enable them to carry out their responsibilities under managed care. Community health psychologists can research, audit, and monitor key performance indicators to assure that managed care is being carried out effectively.

Specific community health psychology activities are organized under the rubrics of managed care education, research, and management. Managed care education includes technical assistance, training and internal marketing activities. Research involves needs analyses to inform internal-external marketing foci, the development of facility assistance plans, and the evaluation of managed care education activities. Management establishes and monitors information concerning the implementation of facility-based managed care. This information is integrated with Research so that appropriate educational and marketing interventions are developed to counter any implementation problems.

The social marketing approach utilizes organizational development (OD) techniques to identify specific needs in the facility and provide technical assistance to help the facility implement effective strategies and overcome barriers that prevent optimum success. The OD approach emphasizes the involvement of all relevant staff in helping to solve the task and using expert consultants only where special knowledge is required (Dannemiller & Jacobs, 1992). Community health psychology plays a "change agent" role in enabling staff to take ownership and promote changes that help to improve service delivery.

With a workforce upon whose shoulders rests the success of providing managed care services to the safety net's patients, the need for internal social marketing is great. For many safety net employees, the implementation of Medicaid Managed Care is seen as one more bureaucratic process, divorced from the real world of interaction with patients. For some staff, it is viewed as an initiative that rewards primary care physicians with salary enhancements or increased status, while creating more burdens for already overworked and less credentialed staff.

There is an identified need for greater support and emphasis on recipient *and* provider education. Provider education is important to motivate physicians to treat patients in a primary care team practice mode that prepays providers at a fixed annual rate. It includes increasing the physicians' motivation to participate in Medicaid Managed Care by delineating its attractive features: having their own panels of patients and families whom they will get to know as they manage all the care patients receive. Primary care physicians also work in teams that assure clinical and administrative supports for providers. Education to properly orient and maintain the relationship between the physicians and the Medicaid Managed Care plan is needed for physicians and their support staff. Education should also include information needed to change provider behavior in managed care plans such as practice guidelines,* goals and objectives, quality assurance requirements and enhanced understanding of the insurance and economic functions of the plan. Such education addresses the important element of controlling cost and quality by cultivating cooperation, providing consistent and responsive feedback, addressing specific problems with providers early, and helping to competitively differentiate safety net Medicaid Managed Care services from private, for-profit Managed Care Organizations (MCOs). However, physicians are not the only group that require internal marketing to make managed care work. Successful managed care requires teamwork, cooperation, changes in role definitions for staff, and even the development of some specialized staff. In addition to staff, managed care must be understood and supported by administrators, community advisory board members, hospital volunteers, and union members. The educational empowerment of all of these participants to create an atmosphere supportive of effectively meeting the needs of consumers through quality delivery of managed care services is critical to success. Education should be directed to inculcating the importance of and imparting techniques for effectively improving the collaboration between all levels of staff, recognizing and strengthening facility-community linkages, integrating

---

*Practice guidelines shape physician behaviors by not reimbursing them if they do not follow the MCO procedures. Further, if physicians *only* performed those practices listed in the guidelines, they will be held harmless for not doing anything else.

care and networking toward satisfying the patient, and making effective and appropriate decisions that foster effective managed care service delivery.

It must be recognized that sustained and repetitive efforts on an organization-wide basis are required to make significant change in a setting as complex as a safety net facility. Evaluation data of how managed care is being implemented, how it is being perceived, and what impact it is having become more than management data. These data become useful for political and marketing purposes.

External marketing involves marketing safety net health services under a single "brand name" in a number of communities. It also involves development, production, and distribution of the health products within its integrated care system in such a manner that consumers—both patients and referring physicians—never have to leave the system to get the health services needed. To accomplish this, the safety net must engage in market research, develop market strategies and tactics, reach consensus on the position facilities should seek to obtain in the market, foster product and personnel changes to implement the strategy, and implement a multi-year advertising and public relations campaign to communicate with the desired markets.

The economic necessity to survive has propelled safety net management into a new world of medical care practice—a world where it has become necessary for all staff to change its "medicocentric culture." The safety net, in embracing the managed care model of service is demonstrating a commitment to provide cost-effective services focused on the primary care needs of the population it serves. However, the fulfillment of this commitment requires a restructuring of the safety net to more clearly focus on managed care, health education, and marketing as core aspects of its mandate. Because of increasing competition, the safety net must increase, in a short time frame, the organizational understanding that *each* employee must assist in the successful management of the patient-customer's perception and expectations. The importance of service excellence in the context of what each employee must do to ensure patient satisfaction necessitates internal marketing to different employee groups and facilities in order to expand the networking options, linkages, and enhanced teamwork that a successful integrated care system demands.

This strategy requires the unprecedented step of involving employees at all levels in a participative planning process that ultimately makes them accountable for maintaining their jobs. Thus, it relates managed care to the process of ongoing continuous quality improvement (CQI)* where a clean environment and courteous staff are as important as high quality health care professionals and expansion and modernization of physical plants in creating a positive experience for patients to use safety net facilities for their health care. Stressing consensus, teamwork, and interdisciplinary participation, community health psychology "coaches" people at different levels to cooperate in solving common problems. The viability of this approach rests on the belief that educating staff to cognitively reframe how they treat patients will enhance the implementation of the managed care model.

A MUNICIPAL HEALTH SYSTEM'S STRATEGIC PLAN

Many states and cities have enacted legislation that reflects the health policy view of managed health care as a possible solution to the problems of increasing expenditures, limited access, and uneven quality within their Medicaid programs. These laws have Medicaid recipients enrolling in managed care[†] plans and being assigned primary care providers who coordinate care and act as gatekeepers[‡] for referrals (Sisk, Gorman, & Carr, 1993). One of their major objectives is to promote preventive medicine, coordinated primary care service delivery, and more rational patterns of medical and health service utilization by Medicaid recipients. New York City began its implementation of managed care plans for its Medicaid population on October 1, 1992. By November 4, 1994, 18 managed care plans were competing with each other to enroll Medicaid patients, with others awaiting state approval. Traditionally, the poor Medicaid recipient was not an attractive market for the voluntary medical sector given lower reimbursement rates for services as compared to other payers and attendant bureaucratic requirements, e.g., more paperwork

---

*Continuous quality improvement refers to a quality improvement process that moves away from the peer review and medical audits implicit in quality assurance to a more positive approach of gradual, unending improvement and setting and achieving ever-higher standards of care.

†Managed care is a system that seeks to control costs by monitoring the delivery of care and limiting access to specialists and costly procedures (Lohman, 1993).

‡Primary care providers are called "gatekeepers" because they manage the care of their patients by coordinating and approving all medical services, laboratory studies, specialty referrals, emergency visits, and hospitalizations (Bellevue Hospital Center, 1993).

(Kwiatkowski & Maislen, 1991). However, in many cases the introduction of managed care for New York State's Medicaid population improved the reimbursement system for service to poor patients. Additionally, as commercial HMO/MCO enrollment has decreased in-patient hospital stays, voluntary hospitals have an increase in empty beds, thus marketing to Medicaid Managed Care patients becomes a way to fill these beds. patients. Consequently many private hospitals began to recruit Medicaid patients away from the nations's largest municipal safety net, the New York City Health and Hospitals Corporation (HHC).

The Mission

HHC understandably felt pressured to "get up to speed" on Medicaid Managed Care quickly. Thus, in March 1993 with little more than an urgent need to stem the increased loss of its major patient revenue base, HHC charged its Office of Primary Care Services with development of a technical training initiative to enable organizational change. Given the prominence of psychologists as executives and administrators within this office, the organizational change agent was to be a newly created Office for Managed Care Education and Special Projects (MCE/SP), directed by the author, a clinical-community psychologist with expertise in cultural diversity training, change management, and community health education. Staff included a doctoral level organizational development behavioral specialist, a doctoral level social psychologist with extensive planning and evaluation skills, and two managers with major administrative coordination, logistics management, and document production skills.

As an operational team, the selected staff brought to their assignment research-and-development, primary-care, mental-health and community-health, human-resources and corporate-training expertise, as well as public-affairs, marketing, information-dissemination, technical-assistance, liaison, and consulting skills. One of our first steps was to diagnose the educational, organizational, administrative, and policy environment in which the training mission was to be met. Specifically, a modified "PRECEDE-PROCEED" model of health promotion planning was utilized to assess some of the *Pre*disposing, *Re*inforcing, and *E*nabling *C*onstructs in the *E*ducational *D*iagnosis and *E*valuation, and the *P*olicy, *R*egulatory, and *O*rganizational *C*onstructs for *E*ducational and *E*nvironmental *D*evelopment of managed care (Green & Kreuter, 1991).

The diagnostic process involved the following elements: definitive statement of the policy and planning issues; identification of the specific issues that concern HHC; researching the past history of the issue, how it first arose and prior attempts to correct it; why it is resurfacing and why past solutions are no longer relevant. Specific questions that required responses were: Who are the present actors involved in the policy/planning issue? What are their relevant strengths and positions on the policy? What are the circumstances or forces which are pushing for a solution to the issue and those which are resisting a change? Given these forces, what are the points of compromise that might lead to a partial or complete solution to the problem? What are the potential feasible solutions and how likely will they be accepted in the light of opposing forces? What form might alternative solutions take?

At the conclusion of the diagnosis, a managed care education plan was put in place that portrayed managed care as a "New Way of Doing Business in Health Care," and an organizational change process was implemented that required each HHC employee to learn how their role ensures customer satisfaction, revenue protection, and the future of HHC. Subsequently, over the course of two fiscal years, managed care education was offered to employees at Central Office and HHC facilities. Training involved the president, Central Office staff, executive directors, affiliation administrators, primary care practitioners, nurses, pharmacists, allied health care staff, and support staff. Board Members and volunteers were also included in the training. The goal of the training was for employees to understand their role and responsibilities under the managed care mode of practice at their facility.

The educational core of the managed care education program is an individually tailored module for different staff groups. These modules are the foundation for training which continues when trainees return to their facilities. Each developed module addresses those employees who have an impact on patient services. The modules provide an interactive learning experience in which employees gain the necessary knowledge base needed to understand managed care and Medicaid Managed Care, and the impact of both on customer service. The information gained in the modules assists employees to successfully manage the customer's perception and expectation. It walks the employee through what happens to a member of a managed care plan from enrollment to accessing the first visit and henceforth. To augment the training, each module also provides various handouts that reinforce learning gained in the training session. These handouts describe the principles of managed care, audience-specific role descriptions, operating procedures, guidelines, processing forms, and other relevant information. Additionally, each module provides scenarios or case studies that allow employees an interactive learning opportunity to experience their new role under managed care.

Unique aspects of these modules, and indeed the total managed care education program, are a commitment to educational empowerment of all the stakeholders in HHC's success or failure and the utilization of social marketing theory and techniques to reach multiple target audiences. Managed care education specifically reaches these audiences by engaging in demographic analysis, telephone surveys, personal interviews, focus groups, service inventories and marketing audits to proceed with the four "Ps" of marketing: Putting the right *product* (managed care) into the right *place* (accessible location) at the right *price* (Medicaid) with the right *promotion*. Such social marketing is particularly informative in assessing what channels can be used to reach target audiences and in suggesting how outcome evaluation can occur. By attending to demographic, cultural, linguistic, and personal characteristics of potential clients, it provides valuable information regarding how to deliver the message, increase attention to the message, enhance its credibility, change negative attitudes, and initiate new behavior patterns. For HHC's diverse patients, this has led to a focus on radio spots and newspaper ads in various languages, personalizing HHC's historic presence in communities of color, and HHC's expertise, trustworthiness, and focus on family care. Evaluation efforts are similarly sensitive to whether all clients have the economic, literacy, or linguistic resources that permit access to them via telephones, questionnaires, or monolingual interviews.

It is important to emphasize that this process differs from past efforts by its particular attention to the implications of managed care for communities of color, how these dovetail with HHC mission and vision, and by its underscoring of issues of change and the environmental, social, and political context of safety net systems and the communities they serve. It serves as an example of how even within highly bureaucratic systems, community health psychologists can mobilize change by reorienting staff behavior toward patients through use of applied behavioral science technology and public health social marketing. Although the proffered empowerment solution primarily serves HHC interests, the creation of a patient-responsive managed care entity also benefits another major stakeholder group, HHC's Medicaid patients, who are primarily persons of color. It represents a change from the inside perspective engineered by a multicultural, multiethnic, and multiracial behavioral scientist-administrator team committed to empowering diverse communities through development of policy, planning, and programs informed by macro issues related to the health care needs of communities of color.

The Issues

In 1994, approximately 60% of HHC's patient base consisted of Medicaid recipients and HHC's market share of over 40% of New York City's Medicaid population accounts for 70% of its revenues (Sheola, 1994; Gibbs, 1993). The strategic planning problem for HHC was how to retain its Medicaid base under state Medicaid reform and how to implement Medicaid Managed Care in a new internal environment in which it must get HHC's Medicaid patient to access its services appropriately so as not to lose money in a capitated payment structure. This case study describes how HHC met this challenge to its fiscal survival in a competitive Medicaid environment while maintaining a public service orientation. It also describes how HHC's Central Office leadership role in managed care policy implementation, oversight, and technical assistance to members of its integrated care network, is evolving from a traditional bureaucratic control style to a consultative and coaching function.

The issue of fulfilling a public trust while adapting to market conditions is important given HHC's creation on July 1, 1970, as a public benefit corporation by the New York State legislature to operate New York City's municipal hospitals (Department of General Services, 1993). HHC's Statement of Purpose emphasizes its determination "as advocate and innovator, to extend equally to all we serve comprehensive health services in an atmosphere of human care and respect" (NYCHHC, 1992). Maintaining this mission in the face of increasing health care expenditures poses a number of policy questions for HHC. Should health service provided at its facilities continue to guarantee equal access to all regardless of ability to pay, be partially paid for by the consumer, of lesser quality or rationed? Should HHC as a semi-autonomous government agency guarantee equality or equity, restrict the patients' freedom or ability to choose providers, be concerned about expenditures or giving quality service to all patients?

These issues are relevant to communities of color with low-income, poor, and uninsured sick residents who have been shunted from private providers to the safety net for uncompensated care. For the negative impact of uncompensated care on HHC's fiscal health can also destabilize the fiscal health of the urban neighborhoods in which HHC hospitals are typically located, since the health care sector is a primary source of jobs in these mainly inner city communities (Coddington, Keen, et al., 1990).

THE IMPORTANCE OF SOCIOPOLITICAL HISTORY

These are not new policy issues for HHC. In fact, HHC was created as a nonprofit health service corporation to establish fiscal autonomy and integrity for the public hospital system and bring the quality of care in the public hospital system up to the standards of the voluntary sector (Pulse Collective, 1990).

In drafting Medicaid and Medicare legislation, Congress failed to accurately envision the entrepreneurial interests of physicians and consequently did not predict their ventures into for-profit institutions, medical laboratories, and new technology expenditures that would contribute to federal deficits. Thus, public safety net institutions like the New York City Department of Hospitals were overwhelmed by those patients who could not pay, afford, or access private care. HHC arose from the vision of major reform in the 1970s zeitgeist encouraging the rise of hospital administration, a discipline which over the next twenty years would limit physicians' control and apply business management concepts to health care.

HHC's history over the past 27 years parallels that of the safety net. Despite attempts to improve fiscal management and public service, HHC hospitals in the 1960s and 1970s continued to be overcrowded, poorly run, viewed by the public as institutions of last resort, and subject to cutbacks in services. In 1972, the control of HHC's board of directors remained with the mayor and its health care service delivery system was a political target for cuts to reduce the city's expenditures. During 1976, three hospitals closed, 10,000 city hospital workers lost their jobs, 3,800 hospital beds were eliminated and major reductions in budgets and services occurred. Critics and supporters alike complained of HHC's poor financial management and planning (Pulse Collective, 1990).

By 1980, Mayor Edward Koch, Congressman Charles Rangel, and the U.S. Secretary of Health and Human Services, crafted a "rescue plan" to stem further hospital closures. Significantly, the plan called for the enrollment of 17,000 low-income East Harlem residents who lacked medical insurance into Citicaid—a pilot HMO.* Matching

---

*A health maintenance organization (HMO) is an insurance plan where for a fixed annual rate all services included in a specific benefit package are provided to the enrollee free or with a copayment at the time of service.

federal funds would be forthcoming if an additional 17,000 patients were enrolled in Medicaid, Medicare, or commercial insurance. The latter would be restricted to only using their insurance at HHC's Metropolitan Hospital, located in Mr. Rangel's East Harlem district.

Subsequently, HHC developed marketing techniques to attract the insured working class and explored other business management strategies: computerized billing, more aggressive collection policies and financial tightening, recruitment of patients with commercial insurance, on-site enrollment of patients in Medicaid, creation of hospital-based group practices, and opening new ambulatory care systems (Pulse Collective, 1990).

Nevertheless, by 1985 HHC served increasingly poorer and sicker patients and was beset by the problems of homelessness, chemical dependency, and AIDS. As HHC's census rose dramatically, its workers' salaries remained fixed, leading to a flight of professional and technical workers from HHC to the voluntary sector. Meanwhile, as nurses and other health workers demanded parity with private hospitals and improved working conditions, new strategies for marketing to the middle class surfaced. In 1987, HHC engaged in a strategic planning* effort and reaffirmed that its mission was to provide for those with no other access to care. In 1989, its board of directors adopted "Strategic Directions" for the year 2000 that involved creation of a community-oriented primary health care system (NYCHHC, 1989).

The 1991 implementation of Medicaid Managed Care in New York State presented HHC with an opportunity to update its strategic plan. It concluded that the 1989 strategic goals remained valid, that progress had been made toward achieving those goals, and it identified follow-up priorities (NYCHHC, 1993c). The update listed the following as key to the implementation of Medicaid Managed Care at HHC; the need to bring HHC up to industry standards by modernization of its physical plant, equipment, and management information System (MIS); projections that there will be continued growth of poverty and of the uninsured in New York City; competition for financially desirable patients leading to a need for attention to bottom-line financial management; and recognition of the then-

---

*Strategic planning requires managers to place their organization in a favorable position in the marketplace. It plays a critical role in providing information about the needs/desires of competitors or other organizations that provide health services, and the general environment in which one must operate—especially what actions government and other third party payers are likely to take (Green & Kreuter, 1991).

current managed competition* discussion and political trends at the federal level. To achieve its goals, HHC concluded that it must both overcome its shortages of primary care providers and aggressively market managed care. A first step was restructuring HHC's financial relationship with the city, such that HHC could maintain a significant portion of the revenue it generated rather than the dollars going into the city's coffers to pay for nonhealth-related budget expenditures. True fiscal autonomy from the city would create economic incentives for HHC managers to reduce inefficiencies and increase productivity, that might lead to salary enhancements and facility improvements. It involved HHC assuming greater risk for budget control as it would no longer have New York City to depend upon exclusively for deficit funding. A restructured HHC-city financial relationship, coupled with New York State's own policy of expanding Medicaid Managed Care, led to a convergence of administrative, political, and economic factors that transformed HHC's Medicaid patient into a consumer with choices. Therefore, HHC's recommitment to its strategic plan both recognized the newly empowered consumer role of its patient and revenue base, and the importance of serving both its sick and healthy constituents with dignity, respect, and humanity.

However, HHC still had to evaluate its strategic planning efforts against the criteria of the characteristics that its future managed care health system must have in order to be sustainable. It has been suggested that assessment criteria for politically viable and workable alternative health care delivery systems, in order of importance, must include: quality of care; universal access; cost stability; minimization of cost shifting; freedom of choice; ease of administration; and financial stability for physicians and hospitals (Coddington et al., 1990).

High quality care from the patient's perspective often includes easy access, individualized attention and caring, and advanced medical technology. The issue here is whether HHC attends to the patient's perspective or actual medical outcomes from a more technical view, which suggest that technology is not necessarily more beneficial than less invasive health care. Universal access is key because of HHC's need to secure compensation for care provided in its public hospitals to the large group of uninsured patients who are often

---

*Managed competition is a system designed to control costs through competition, not price controls. Organized groups of doctors and other practitioners, hospitals, insurers, and HMOs compete for customers by offering standardized packages (Lohman, 1993).

turned away by for-profit providers. Cost stability must be achieved since the middle class and the city are increasingly dissatisfied with the escalating proportion of their budgets and tax bills which support health care expenditures. Cost shifting,* which leads to an unfair allocation of uncompensated health care costs to safety net providers, negatively impacts the competitiveness of HHC.

In concert, the above became the considerations that HHC included in deciding what actions to take in implementing Medicaid Managed Care. It also had to consider a key provision of the Statewide Managed Care Act, which mandated local social services departments to participate in managed care systems to the extent that by 1993, 10%, by 1995, 25%, and by 1997, 50% of New York City's Medicaid population not exempt or excluded from participation[†] must be enrolled in such plans (New York State Department of Social Services [NYSDDS], 1993).

---

*Cost shifting occurs when cost to a particular payer is raised to offset losses incurred by providing services to other groups. It means that those who can, pay more, to offset the cost of care for those who cannot pay enough or at all.

[†]Previously exclusion from participation in Medicaid Managed Care systems was granted to Medicaid recipients who: were receiving services from a residential health care facility, long-term home care program, hospice, state hospital for the mentally ill, residential treatment facility for children or youth, inpatient institution operated by the Veteran's Administration; had a chronic infirmity, condition, or disability; were receiving services from a certified home health agency, and had medical needs which were more appropriately met outside of the managed care program; were enrolled in an HMO under a health insurance program other than Medicaid or another managed care program authorized by the New York State Department of Social Services. *Exemption* from mandatory enrollment can be requested by Medicaid recipients who meet the following criteria: No managed care provider is located to afford them reasonable access to service; they reside in a temporary shelter or home; they have an established relationship with a nonparticipating PCP for at least one year and have seen that PCP more than three times in the past year (the period may be less than one year for a pregnant woman who has been receiving ongoing prenatal care/services from the PCP); they cannot be served by a managed care participating provider because of language barriers, and have an established relationship, as previously defined, with a PCP who speaks their language; or are receiving special care (mental health, alcohol or substance abuse services) on more than an incidental base and are under the care of a special care provider. Such exemptions are under attack by Republican/Conservative majorities in New York and other states, and have been or are gradually being discontinued in New York and elsewhere.

Given HHC's treatment of nearly half of the city's Medicaid patients, it appears to have little choice but to attach tremendous importance to the fiscal implications of each of the criteria. In its favor is the fact that HHC is ideally suited for managed care with all components of a managed health care system under its corporate umbrella. With participation in Medicaid Managed Care, HHC also stands to make further progress in attaining its goals of delivering community-oriented primary health care (Carrillo, 1991).

PERSPECTIVES OF DIFFERENT PLAYERS

The current actors involved in the implementation of Medicaid Managed Care at HHC are its patients, health care providers, employees, and administrators. There are other players including economists, insurers, politicians, and state and city officials,* but their roles are less direct than the former groups which have higher stakes in the successful implementation of managed care at HHC. Not surprisingly, each actor has diverse positions on the policy and the planning procedures in operationalizing Medicaid Managed Care at HHC. Additionally, not all actors are as equally well-organized and this impacts on how effective each will be in having their and the patient's concerns addressed. Finally, often there is not even an intergroup homogeneity of positions. Indeed, one of the most important actors—the patient—more often than not witnesses how other actors attempt to speak on his or her behalf. Bearing these considerations in mind, what follows is an attempt at assessing the relevant strengths and positions of the major players toward identifying what HHC viewed as potentially feasible solutions to its planning concerns.

Patients

Entrepenueurial supporters of managed care and competition wish to believe that patients are able to operate in the health care market with the same "buyer beware" caution they bring to other purchases when they are *well informed* about their choices. Thus, they are viewed as clients, consumers, or customers.

However, physician critics suggest that there is no incentive for Medicaid patients to act like consumers since they are insulated

---

*HHC's senior administrators are city officials who respond to the demands of the city's highest elected politician—the mayor.

from the influencing factor of costs by the government's role as payer. Additionally, some acutely ill patients often face life or death concerns in making informed decisions about health care that can lead to noneconomical choices being made (Relman, 1993). Also, sick or worried patients may not be inclined to stay in a managed care plan, and may seek care not covered by the plan that is perceived as the best, and the price is secondary. Patients are also heavily dependent on the advice and judgment of health professionals, who often decide what type of health services they need.

In response to critics and reported Medicaid Managed Care marketing abuses and deceptive enrollment practices in which some managed care organizations have engaged in capturing the Medicaid patient, city and state governments have begun to mandate that specific information be provided to patients and to conduct random audits of all plan enrolled members.

Communities: Cultural versus structural views

Some critics subscribe to the belief that HHC's Medicaid patients, who are by and large from ethnic, racial, and class groups historically underserved by private enterprise systems, will suffer from the rationing of care provided under a managed care system. To buttress this perspective, they indicate that increased access for the urban poor (who are generally sicker than the nonpoor and have many unmet health care needs such as AIDS and tuberculosis) (Ehrenreich, 1990) is necessary to achieve improved health rather than restricting access to care for this population. Rather than viewing the consumer as empowered by managed care plans, some critics question the further entrepreneurial empowerment of "big business" involved in the delivery of managed care services (McNamee, 1993).

The issue of how social class, race, and ethnicity are assumed to limit access to medical care is pivotal in terms of planning how to use limited resources for implementation of Medicaid Managed Care. The usual explanations for the inverse relationship states that poor, ethnically and racially diverse patients are less likely to utilize health services because of a culture of poverty or other cultural deficit in health knowledge, attitude, or behavior, and social structural arrangements. The cultural view states that the culture of such patients does not place a high value on health and that though this lesser appreciation may have originally been based on economic deprivation, it has taken on a functional autonomy that is transmitted intergenerationally. This perspective has been critiqued for its victim-blaming ideology by numerous policy analysts and psychologists in particular (Ryan, 1976; De La Cancela, 1986, 1989b).

The structural view alternatively examines the context of care or the characteristics of health systems to which different groups have access. Many low income people are not eligible for Medicaid, nor for Medicaid Managed Care, and are likely to receive uncompensated care in the public hospitals' clinics and emergency rooms, where care is often impersonal and dehumanized. Additional problems of inadequate transportation in poor neighborhoods, inconvenient clinic hours and long waits, lack of ongoing relationships with primary care providers, and a curative orientation and specialist focus on the part of physicians lead to further deterrent effects on care seekers. The culprit here is the culture of medicine rather than the culture of the individual patient or community. Medicocentric culture consists of the habits, customs, and expectations of health professionals and the bureaucracies for which they work. Proponents of the structural perspective suggest providing patients with a "good" experience in HHC facilities by changing professional and organizational behavior to culturally competent, preventive, and community-based services (Ortiz, 1993). Cultural competence is a system of care that is sensitive to culture at all levels: practice, governance, and policy. It requires a *measurable* capacity to *function* effectively with varied social groups (De La Cancela, Jenkins, & Chin, 1993).

Combining organizational, psychological, and health education analyses focuses attention on managed care as a systematic attempt to change the behavior of both providers and Medicaid clients through a series of incentives and requirements. The critical concern is how Medicaid patients will fare within managed care plans that accept capitation* payments, which contain a financial incentive for providers to provide fewer services. Along these lines HHC, together with other safety net providers, educates its Medicaid patients to stay within their system of care. In fact, HHC pledged to undergo an organizational culture shift to have patients use their services out of choice rather than necessity (Cooper, 1993). HHC's marketing as a provider of choice speaks of patient satisfaction and customer service while simultaneously emphasizing that its workforce mirrors the community and HHC's social contract of service to diverse linguistic and cultural groups (NYCHHC, 1993b).

---

*Capitation is a fixed, predetermined monthly payment to providers that covers all contracted services for HMO members in advance. Providers agree to provide specified services to members for a specified length of time, regardless of how often they use the services (De La Cancela et al., 1993).

Providers: Health care professionals

Given capitation's predictable reimbursements and financial incentives to provide fewer services, the perspective of some health care providers has changed from a historic reluctance to accept the lower reimbursement rates (in comparison to Medicare and private insurance patients) for services rendered to a more favorable view of Medicaid payments (Cornelius, 1991). However, critics within the health provider community have questioned the benefit of market values on medical services. They argue that the relationship between physicians and patients should be substantially different than that between entrepreneur and customer (Relman, 1992). Doctors are expected to be altruistic and committed to patient care, acting as advocates and counselors in the best interests of the patient. Yet, the recent deprofessionalization of the medical sector and the commercialization of health care have led doctors to be more interested in the economic operation of lucrative medical practices that provide opportunities for additional income.

The rise of a "medical industrial complex" or corporatization of health care has occurred, in which nonprofit and public hospitals are forced to compete with investor-owned hospitals and a rapidly growing network of for-profit ambulatory facilities. Consequently, voluntary and public hospitals experience themselves as beleaguered businesses and act accordingly, using advertising, marketing, and public relations techniques to attract more patients. Illustrative is HHC's sales training to promote enrollment in its HMO. Additionally, the government is more encouraging of competition and free markets in medicine, believing both will limit expenditures. In fact, while privatization of health care is being suggested, some are wary given a belief that health care flourishes best in the private sector *with* public support to meet its societal responsibilities, avoiding dominance by business interests. Some physicians are concerned about possible conflicts of interest and their ability to make decisions that determine what medical services will be provided in each case, and thus to determine the aggregate expenditures for health care. Therefore, they advise that the medical profession and society must reaffirm their de facto social contract to serve the needs of the sick. They also warn that any proposed health care reform will not be successful without a properly motivated medical profession. In their opinion, a greater reliance on group practice and on medical insurance, which prepays providers at a fixed annual rate, offers the best chance of solving the economic problems of health care. They further state that most problems can be well handled, and at less expense, by generalist physicians (Relman, 1993).

HHC physicians also see themselves as key to the implementation of Medicaid Managed Care at HHC. HHC recognizes the strengths of generalist physicians in the gatekeeper role and has sought to hasten implementation of Medicaid Managed Care by requesting and receiving $25 million from the City of New York toward increasing the number of primary care physicians and enhancing primary care attending salaries.* The funding was also utilized to add other professional staff such as registered nurses, nurse's aides, social workers, Health Educators, quality assurance coordinators, and other ancillary health staff. HHC has sought to motivate these providers to become more customer service oriented in the provision of care by taking the customer's perspective in designing managed care programs and placing a high priority on customer satisfaction.

Yet, some HHC health care providers have voiced skepticism regarding HHC's ability to meet the challenge of motivating them to successfully implement managed care. In part, the professional staff concerns centered around the issue of equitable salaries for all providers whose history of public service to the city's poor and underserved was not adequately recognized by HHC's then current exclusion of nurse practitioners, psychiatrists, and other physician specialists from the official HHC designation of Primary Care Attending.

Other aspects of their skepticism relate to assessments bred by service in a municipal hospital system whose bureaucracy is not impervious to political pressures and the budget policies and priorities of a mayor committed to exploring the privatization of hospitals, a system struggling to maintain its service infrastructure given a history of being undercapitalized, a system used as a dumping ground by private hospitals that seek to avoid or to limit service to the poor (Pulse Collective, 1990). Additionally, HHC health care providers as a group are more aligned with a liberal and, in some cases, progressive tradition of health care practice, yet they are generally the products of a professional socialization process that makes them wary of

---

*Primary care attendings agreed to minimally provide six office sessions per week, one of them in the evening or weekend, scheduled appointments for routine and walk-in visits, 24-hour phone coverage, and admitting privileges in the appropriate clinical service. They work in teams with nurses, social workers, and other providers to provide comprehensive care to their panel of patients. Primary care providers (PCPs) must be Board certified or eligible in internal medicine, pediatrics, obstetrics/gynecology, or family practice.

the threat of greater government control on their autonomous practices, expertise, and authority. Rather than Medicaid Managed Care, many of HHC's physicians emphasize the need for more primary care doctors, protection from the threat of violence in the neighborhoods in which HHC facilities are located, and the need to teach patients who have become dependent upon emergency rooms how to participate in traditional care (Rosenthal, 1993).

Providers: Institutional service associations

Health care providers as a group, especially physicians, wield considerable influence in HHC and any other safety net facility because they are prominent in the communities served and are adept at political lobbying. Thus, their relative strength compared to that of unorganized patients is considerable. In this regard, HHC recognizes that the American Medical Association has a long history of opposition to a series of health care reform proposals, including national health insurance and universal coverage through a single payer system (Pear, 1993). Yet within the world of managed care at HHC, hospitals and D&TCs* are also "providers" or entities that provide or arrange for the provision of services for Medicaid recipients enrolled in a managed care program, such that discussion of the providers' relative strengths and positions must include the organizational views of those provider associations of which HHC hospitals and neighborhood family care centers are members.

The American Hospital Association (AHA) sees leadership as the key to successful transformation of the health care delivery system. Thus, it is developing tools for educating hospital leadership (CEOs, board members, doctors) to the changes in organizational values and culture required to integrate into new systems (Fraser & Tappert, 1993). One key question to be addressed is how hospitals and networks can overcome internal and external barriers to patient-centered care so that they can coordinate service across provider sites. AHA members believe that the changes require internal restructuring of facilities, strengthening linkages between facilities, and developing and participating in community networks with other private and public networks (Ferguson, 1993). Their suggested reform strategies include: the development of community-based pri-

---

*Diagnostic and treatment center (D&TC) is a freestanding facility certified under public health law engaged principally "in providing services by or under the supervision of a physician for the prevention, diagnosis or treatment of human disease, pain, injury, deformity or physical condition."

mary care and prevention oriented clinics; expansion of existing community clinics in high need areas; and coalition building with private hospitals, community health centers, government, philanthropy, business, academia, and the broader community.

These are strategies that HHC has already utilized; in particular, HHC has exerted leadership in founding Action for Primary Care Legislation, a broad statewide coalition of organizations and individuals interested in developing and assuring access to high quality, comprehensive primary care services for all New Yorkers (Action for Primary Care Legislation, 1993). As such, HHC has committed itself to looking beyond Medicaid Managed Care coverage to cure the symptoms of its ailing health care system, recognizing that Medicaid Managed Care plans, while responsive to current economic trends, are not panaceas. Thus, it has agreed to pursue the retraining of its existing labor force as well as the retooling of health care education programs to develop an appropriate primary care system. This involves redesigning physician residency training programs to provide hands-on experience at community sites. It also involves hiring patient educators and health educators to be available in the emergency department (ED) of facilities participating in Medicaid Managed Care. These educators will serve as counselors who can personally explain to nonurgent patients inappropriately seeking services in the ED the proper procedures and benefits of accessing services through Medicaid Managed Primary Care. Specifically, patient health educators will emphasize how HHC has implemented health system changes that make their neighborhood primary care sites or D&TCs more user-friendly through extended hours of operation including evenings and weekends. For those not enrolled in managed care, patient educators can help them register for Medicaid if eligible, and connect them to representatives of HHC's HMO, MetroPlus if interested.

HHC also increases access to community-based primary care through Communicare, a program targeting families in 13 medically underserved neighborhoods. Communicare is available to all patients regardless of their ability to pay and does not require enrollment in an HMO or other managed care plan. However, it does follow the Medicaid Managed Care model of practice by assigning each patient a primary care doctor who will coordinate and monitor their health care needs (Chu, 1993). It is intended that the Communicare sites provide the same level of service from health promotion to tertiary care to all patients including indigent service, as do all of HHC facilities (Bellevue Hospital Center, 1993). The objective of the Communicare program is to maximize service delivery to the poor and in that vein help them register for Medicaid if eligible and access a managed care plan. Communicare also funds health educators to teach patients how to utilize HHC's primary care system most efficaciously (Nathanson, 1993).

The National Association of Community Health Centers takes the position that it is critical that any health care reform, whether national or state based, assure that essential health care providers, such as health centers, disproportionate share hospitals, and public health agencies are adequately reimbursed and protected for care provided to those currently enrolled in Medicaid and those currently uninsured. Thus, along with HHC and other safety net providers, it calls for state Medicaid programs to explicitly recognize the costs of providing extra care, such as social services for the homeless as well as transportation and translation for the poor or linguistically diverse (NYCHHC, 1993b).

Significantly, community health center advocates call attention to the importance of public agencies to position themselves to compete in a private arena, the barriers in accomplishing this without data and feedback from the communities served, and the need to be responsive to the needs of a diverse population and how these can be met through use of mid-level providers* and behavioral health professionals. Their views are relevant to community health psychology given a shared view of public policy responsibility and the need for environmental, social, and political analysis of where different provider associations' interests can be complementary or antagonistic to the populations' needs. Illustrative are the views of some: orthopaedic surgeons opposed to appropriately trained podiatrists performing leg surgery; psychiatrists against properly trained health service psychologist providers receiving prescription privileges; and opthamalogists insisting that optometrists be limited to use of a formulary of pre-approved drugs. These arguments and similar calls in the recent past for exclusion of these competent and qualified professionals from hospital staff and clinical privileges, managed care panels, and Medicaid/Medicare reimbursement are often related to the guild and economic interests of the opposing medical specialists.

However, the issues for patients are ones of benefits to the public's access to comprehensive health care, especially in rural populations and underserved urban locales and in recognition that each of these professions, along with certified advanced nurse clinicians, have a history of providing cost-effective community health center services to the poor and underserved.

---

*Mid-level providers refers to nonphysician health care professionals such as nurse practitioners, physician assistants, and nurse midwives.

ORGANIZATIONAL RESISTANCE TO CHANGE

With a workforce of approximately fifty thousand, HHC is a super-agency whose health care economy provides a major source of jobs that often overworks, understaffs, ill-equips, and underpays its workers. This reality is not due to some organized malevolence on the part of HHC administrators. It is, however, intimately related to the health expenditure crisis that places many public hospitals in a precarious existence as they serve the poor. With the arrival of Medicaid Managed Care and the current health competition climate, HHC employees are being asked to embrace health care reform while significant numbers of them wonder if they are just being asked to do more with less resources, economic and otherwise, under the guise of reform.

For many employees, the implementation of Medicaid Managed Care is one more bureaucratic mandate, responsive to the needs of HHC's central office but divorced from the employees' highly-charged daily interaction with patients at the facilities. For others, the fear is that a second tier of care will be provided to patients. Some feel that most doctors, nurses, other clinicians, and administrators have professional distancing "attitudes" that lead them to treat patients in routine and impersonal ways. Finally, there are those who state that the demands for care at HHC already exceed supply, that budget cuts will continue, and that it is difficult to retain and recruit staff given HHC's vulnerability to political pressures.

In June 1993, HHC's Office of Primary Care Services and Alternative Delivery Systems (OPCS) assessed its strengths, weaknesses, opportunities and threats (SWOTS) during a strategic planning retreat organized to further its goals and mission. The analysis revealed that the department's management, professional, and support staff experienced its strengths as being: diversified educational and work backgrounds; commitment to HHC's mission; teamwork; enthusiasm for primary care services; and hard work and dedication. Weaknesses were: not enough professional staff; heavy workloads making it difficult to keep track of multiple assignments; delays in hiring support staff; antiquated computer systems; lack of communication between all staff; lack of staff involvement in decision making; and lack of cohesion between offices within HHC.

Opportunities were perceived to be: accomplishment of something that had not been done before; having the lead role in the implementation of managed care; training facility staff on operational issues; high visibility on the local and national level; and being able to work with individuals who are well respected and knowledgeable in the field. Identified threats were: limited acceptance of managed care among HHC professionals and patients; difficulty of changing staff and patient behavior regarding managed care; inability to tell facilities how to implement managed care; inability to develop staff; lack of positive communication and feedback; and fiscal, political, and time pressures and constraints (NYCHHC, 1993d). The results of the SWOTS study revealed that senior staff and administrative support staff were concerned about HHC's institutional resistance to change, and felt that educational empowerment of all levels of HHC staff was necessary to make Medicaid Managed Care work. They felt strongly that their initiatives were dependent upon the cooperation of HHC staff to be trained and implement what is learned. A necessary component was to ensure that all levels of staff understand managed care and, particularly, their roles in carrying out effective and efficient multidisciplinary teamwork and coordination.

Environmental Analysis

HHC has an annual operating budget in excess of $3.8 billion. Its major sources of income are Medicaid revenues from the city, state and federal governments totaling approximately $2.1 billion in fiscal year 1993, and $1.9 billion in fiscal year 1994 and comprising 70% of its budget (Sheola, 1994; Cook & Webb, 1993). HHC's Medicaid Managed Care restructuring began in July 1992. Yet recent reports on the state of New York City hospitals warn that it stands to lose significant amounts of this revenue if it cannot compete adequately for patients (G. Scott, 1993; United Hospital Fund [UHF], 1993). While HHC has made important strides, deficiencies must be addressed in the area of staff shortages, low salaries, staff burnout, insufficient training, and limited educational opportunities. HHC serves patients who tend to have relatively complex health care needs at facility locations that many consider undesirable (UHF, 1993). HHC must find ways to attract and retain patients who now have other options.

The City Hospital Visiting Committee, a watchdog agency, reports that HHC's efforts to enroll patients in managed care requires recruiting additional providers to decrease waiting times for primary care appointments. Attaining this objective also requires increased patient education and cultural competence in patient education and in delivery of services in order to increase responsiveness to community needs. Additionally, recognition that patients, given their options to go elsewhere, must be satisfied suggests that HHC must engage in more social marketing, community outreach, and patient follow up. The same tier of service has to be provided to patients who are ineligible for or whose medical needs are best met outside of Medicaid Managed Care (UHF, 1993).

Similar to what occurred in recent discussions regarding the need for health care reform, most of the involved actors agree on the need to move ahead with planning for the implementation of Medicaid Managed Care (Clymer, 1993). Not surprisingly, however, labor, doctors, nurses, hospitals, and patients all differ over how to implement Medicaid Managed Care. All of these constituencies insist on having their needs met in whatever process emerges. These groups are likely to influence HHC to retain its Medicaid base while maintaining a public service orientation. How this balance is established will depend upon how each group empowers itself to participate in HHC's implementation of Medicaid Managed Care.

The Alternatives: Enrollee-provider education

In New York State's annual report on Medicaid Managed Care, the Department of Social Services identified a need for greater support and emphasis on recipient and provider education activities (NYSDSS, 1993) Although these efforts are likely to be time-consuming, labor intensive, and expensive, the state emphasizes that recipients must understand the nature of managed care, its advantages and limitations, and that throughout the course of their enrollment, these managed care principles must be reinforced. The report states that it is crucial to reinforce the appropriate behavior of Medicaid Managed Care patients because they do not have the disincentive of paying for any unauthorized service use.

Herein lies one alternative for HHC to pursue to ensure the success of Medicaid Managed Care: maintaining policies and procedures regarding enrollee education, as per the State Department of Social Services (DSS) requirements. Such education would be an ongoing process to include in concert with health maintenance and illness prevention efforts: orientation to provider services, instruction in self-management of medical problems, a written patients' bill of rights, appropriate use of the referral system, grievance procedures, after-hours coverage system, and provisions for emergency treatment. Additionally, health education literature on personal health care behavior and care, breast self-examination, prevention/testing for HIV and other sexually transmitted diseases, pap smear testing, tuberculosis, lead poisoning, asthma, family planning, vision and hearing testing, prenatal care, fetal alcohol syndrome, well child care (including immunizations), parenting, hypertension screening, cancer screening, nutritional guidance, smoking cessation, alcohol and drug dependency and weight management should be readily available and accessible to all enrollees through their primary care provider or primary care team members, e.g., nurse, health educator, or social worker, and to potential enrollees through HHC health fairs, community events, and facility information tables. Linguistically appropriate education is also required; once 10% or 500 Medicaid Managed Care plan members in a borough are identified as primarily using a language other than English, all materials must be translated—this includes braille or audio tapes for the blind.

The importance of enrollee education is likely to be accepted by most of the actors involved in planning Medicaid Managed Care implementation at HHC because of its emphasis on helping the enrollee to appropriately use the managed care plan. It has the advantage of already being a contractual requirement for provider participation in the state's Medicaid reform effort, and thus, is a contractual responsibility that can be transferred to participating provider groups and monitored by HHC's HMO, MetroPlus. Another benefit is that it builds on the orientation and introduction to Medicaid Managed Care Services that the state is already providing in local social service district Income Support Centers. An educated consumer is empowered to get the individualized attention available to which she is entitled in a primary care setting. Education also has the benefit of ensuring that HHC providers and hospitals receive the benefits of lower costs since inappropriate access to care is aggressively discouraged. In essence, education makes the patient a well-informed consumer with knowledge of the choices available to her. A patient education and outreach program is a cost-effective way to teach Medicaid Managed Care enrollees how to use the system appropriately (Herrick, 1993). The goals of such a program are to inform the Medicaid Managed Care enrollees of their health care choices and to assist them in choosing the best program to meet their needs, help control costs, and improve outcomes.

The same can be said of provider education, which motivates physicians to treat patients in a primary care team practice model that prepays providers at a fixed annual rate, and which is reinforced by HHC's payment of enhanced salaries for agreeing to participate in Medicaid Managed Care. Provider education for physicians and their office staff also properly orients and maintains the relationship between the physicians and the Medicaid Managed Care plan (Kongstvedt, 1993b, 1993a). This alternative highlights the importance of HHC's investing in provider education and re-education because it is one of the common omissions of managed health care plans. This failure may lead to the improper use by physicians of authorization systems, providing or promising services that the plan does not cover, or allowing open-ended authorizations to specialists. Such improper use defeats the cost-effective gatekeeper role and policy of providing services based on authorization from the HMO, and reducing inappropriate access to specialists who traditionally admit patients to costly hospitalization.

In essence, this first alternative deals with the challenge of managed care in two ways: first, by concentrating on patients empowered through education, and second, by giving a professional group of employees, doctors, the education and incentives they need to promote this change. However, this strategy does not address the understandable suspicion of staff and institutional resistance to change* that the implementation of Medicaid Managed Care can promote within HHC. Thus, another alternative can be chosen to convert HHC into a patient-oriented managed care entity.

Organizational Development

HHC's second alternative is targeting its educational efforts and marketing to a broader group that includes providers, employees, administrators, executive directors, consumers, community advisory boards, union members, critics, and supporters. This approach focuses on organizational development,[†] social marketing, and large-scale event technology, an interactive planning strategy of increasing all stakeholder's ownership of and commitment to changes, in HHC's way of doing business and services delivery (Dannemiller & Jacobs, 1992).

Rather than solely relying on the thinly disguised "blaming the victim" perspective in which patient education is provided to Medicaid recipients to overcome their "cultural deficits" in health access behavior or attitude, large-scale technology[‡] involves a struc-

---

*Institutional resistance refers to the myriad organizational dynamics that predispose staff to fear and mistrust change from the status quo, e.g., rumors, power cliques and solo practice rather than teamwork.

†Organizational development utilizes behavioral science theory and technology and involves long-term planned change strategies.

‡Large-scale technology utilizes an action research approach for activities such as training and human resources development. Applied to managed care education, it recognizes that managed care is attempting to intervene within an established sociotechnical system where staff and patients have learned to survive and to meet needs in spite of conditions that outsiders might view as unsatisfactory (Gunatilake & Forouzesh, 1989–90). Thus, personal relationships and influences, internal interaction and relationships, and external forces are assessed through involvement of internal and external stakeholders in developing and implementing managed care administrative processes, procedures, education, and marketing.

tural analysis of the patient's health access behavior and the providers' "culture of medicine" to reveal what aspect of care at HHC needs to change. A core principle of this diagnostic effort is identifying and reducing defensiveness, among all stakeholders, including patients, workers, and administrators, thereby setting a new organizational norm that blaming others for problems is no longer acceptable (Dannemiller & Jacobs, 1992). Another key practice is educational empowerment, which requires humanizing and personalizing care, and changing the habits, customs, and expectations of health providers (whether they are health care professionals or bureaucracies) to become more consumer-focused, outcome-oriented, and value based. The implications of this paradigm shift* are a true recognition of the cultural diversity of both HHC's patients and workforce, as well as a wider definition of how HHC seeks to involve the community of internal and external consumers it serves. Empowerment here refers to both clarifying what the incentives are for participation in this new mode of service delivery and delineation of where the accountability for its success lies and what is required to achieve it.

This alternative involves the use of ongoing interactive strategic planning, institutional "coaching," total quality management, and functional training sessions, targeted to over 58 key staff groups. All of these activities utilize applied behavioral science practices, networking, and community health educational theories to reach large groups of people in a short period of time. The interactive nature of the experience is reflected in the sessions attending to the perspectives of all of the participant groups to "co-create the process" for implementation of managed care at HHC that is well suited to its public service mission. A key component of this technology involves the identification of how staff, employees, volunteers, administrators, and providers are consumers of each others' services within the larger organization. Internally, these groups are each others' clients and customers, as patients, their families, vendors, and community members assume these roles externally. The intent here is to emphasize the need for coordination of services, the recognition and strengthening of linkages, and networking toward satisfying the patient—the ultimate client, consumer, customer.

---

*Paradigm shift refers to a change in organizational perspective or conceptual framework from which environmental and institutional conditions are interpreted and managed (Wilkenfeld, 1994).

Such an approach reassures employees that HHC has abandoned neither the patient nor the employee. In fact, it taps into their commitment to the HHC mission, encourages new quality teams, provides them with skills to improve collaboration between all levels of staff, and, most importantly, involves them in decision making. The purpose and process of each educational, training, and marketing activity and how it fits into the large picture of HHC's future is explained clearly to participants. The process calls for ongoing input from physicians, hospitals, and consumers through participation in education design teams and workgroups in response to changes in the internal and external environment of HHC (Elmhurst Hospital Center, 1993). This human resource development approach supplements the resource planning, financial and facility planning in which HHC must continue to engage, by building up organizational skills for employees to motivate each other, and developing good working relationships with other health professionals, paraprofessionals, Medicaid recipients, Medicaid Managed Care enrollees, and patients. The approach is a workplace education program aimed at re-orienting staff in their behavior towards patients and each other through use of consumer psychology, health communication techniques, and education for critical action (empowerment).

For example, in designing managed care functional training,* employees are consulted by managers about how to carry out their roles under managed care. This imparts the message that informed employees have the capability to perform their roles, will accept responsibility for carrying them out and benefit from evaluation and feedback to improve productivity and quality. From such involvement, training manuals for participant use are created that include: background information about the Medicaid Managed Care plan and managed care concepts in general; primary care provider responsibilities, description of the functions of other departments, e.g., quality assurance, billing, authorization, and other plan policies and procedural requirements; and review of benefits. These manuals can be used for both self-study and with trainers who are themselves from the employee groups being trained at a particular session (MacLeod, 1994). Most importantly, these manuals reinforce the need to have a customer service orientation, reminding

---

*Functional training refers to extensive group experiential learning that allows large numbers of individuals from various facilities and organizational levels to examine how their job roles, responsibilities, and goals need to change in response to a changing service delivery environment.

staff that if HHC provides poor customer service, there are many other providers who are now willing and happy to service HHC's patients.

The acceptance of this second alternative is high because its goal is to shift participants from turf-related competition to open communication and collaboration. It is attractive because it does not limit involvement to a small team of planners and thus avoids limiting the resources of experience and reducing the level of commitment to implement Medicaid Managed Care. In synchronicity with HHC's strategic plan, this alternative creates more effective cross-functional working relationships by involving internal and external customers, line managers, and front line workers throughout the planning process. These participants act as constant "reality checks" on how faithful HHC is to its mission (Dannemiller & Jacobs, 1992).

EMPOWERMENT THROUGH EDUCATION

An educational empowerment strategy was selected as the preferred way to promote a viable organizational response to the need for maintaining and improving the quality of integrated patient focused services provided by HHC. The selected large-scale event technology was one in which key HHC personnel were taught, first by expert consultants and then by the Office of Managed Care Education and Special Projects (MCE/SP) to conduct training for mixed multi-facility groups of up to 200 staff of all levels. MCE/SP utilized data-based monitoring to identify how the selected personnel were faring in the development and implementation of facility-based large-scale events. Additionally, we conducted needs analyses among HHC stakeholders to identify the areas in which consultation, technical assistance, and marketing strategies were necessary. Specifically, we conducted telephone and mail surveys, individual interviews of key informants (staff, providers, physicians), and focus groups with eight target audiences* to secure in-depth reaction to the large-scale events or elements of an event.

Simultaneously, we developed close relationships with the managed care coordinators of all HHC facilities to identify other key staff who might both assist in identification of differences in consumer

---

*Groups included: clerks; managed care coordinators; finance and MIS staff; risk management/quality assurance; allied health care; nursing; nurse practitioners/midwives; and physicians.

health attitudes, beliefs, behavior, knowledge, and desires as regards managed care, and who might be appropriate nominees for selection as internal facilitators* to expand the trainer pool. Informed by these efforts, by September 1993 we had developed final drafts of areas and issues the educational curriculum should encompass, and identified and trained a group of a hundred internal facilitators through a nomination and application process that granted a symbol of accomplishment, prestige, and status as managed care ambassador to those selected. We also developed a Likert-type questionnaire that generally assessed what perceptions, knowledge, attitudes, and beliefs regarding managed care existed in the target population pre-training and post-intervention.

Space does not permit an extensive delineation of all of the behavioral determinants extant among the target HHC staff audiences that the educational diagnosis identified, thus a few positive and negative factors will be presented to highlight the contributions of the PRECEDE model. Some negative predisposing factors were lack of knowledge of managed care or misinformation; lack of confidence in being able to adapt to managed care and fear of what managed care meant; and perceived lack of autonomy in the workplace and deference to health care professionals. Positive predisposing factors included a wish for independence, and desire and ability to advocate for oneself. Negative enabling factors included limited meeting space in facilities sufficiently large to hold up to 200 people at a time. Positive enablers were provision of communication abilities and general interest in educational programming. Positive reinforcers were health care providers committed to encouraging patients to practice preventive health behaviors and to be more independent health consumers. Negative reinforcement existed in institutional racism, sexism, classism and biased beliefs, attitudes, behaviors, and images that served as barriers to communication across cultures, among health personnel, and in the practitioner-patient encounter.

A team of psychologists, health educators, health care program planners, analysts, consultants, managers, and public health and public administration externs utilized behavioral science principles to develop a positive response to the organizational crisis engendered by managed care. Thus, a crisis with profound emotional im-

---

*Internal facilitators were selected by the following criteria: nomination by peers; endorsement by executive director and department manager; previous training/education experience; public speaking/presentation skills; front line rather than leadership role; and job title expertise.

plications for staff at varied levels was identified: the loss of identity and the sense of being grounded when workers lose their customary roles, comfort, and familiarity with the old way of "doing business"; grief related to the perceived loss of specialty status, earned through years of education, residency, and experience, given managed care's emphasis on and valuing of "generalist" primary Care practitioners; and resentment toward HHC and its administrators for "rewarding" others with salary enhancements while they are being "punished."

These feelings, beliefs, expectations, and behaviors contribute to stress, anxiety, uncertainty, and ambiguity about what organizational change is going to mean for staff on a daily basis (Wilkenfeld, 1994). Psychosocial-behavioral variables can contribute to employees leaving the organization if they cannot develop adequate coping skills to handle these emotions. Thus, the paradigm shift to which HHC committed itself had to also provide tools for staff at all levels to find the opportunity in the health care crisis they encounter. This requires cognitive reframing* on the individual level, examining personal mission statements and goals as employees and health personnel in light of HHC's objective to provide managed care. Thus, the developed educational curriculum provides support, understanding, and the emotional climate to allow participants to explore their own feelings and thoughts about managed care, and to redefine relationships and find new ways to collaborate with each other.

An enabling educational program was designed for staff and providers to develop understanding, motivation, and skills to reduce the risks managed care poses to HHC and its external consumers. Participants were encouraged to involve themselves more proactively in their facility's preparation for managed care. The educational program specifically focused on empowerment and voluntary, active, participative learning to reduce suspicions and resistance to "training."

Given previous human resources experiences some staff view HHC-provided training as propaganda, politically or commercially directed, or paternalistic. Instead the MCE/SP educational modules nurtured an increased awareness mentality within the context of participants' daily work and its intersection with social, economic, and health policies. Educational empowerment assisted in the development of participants' self-confidence and promoted a sense of

---

*Cognitive reframing refers to individual shifts in perspective and the process of thinking about things from a different point of view or set of beliefs/values.

efficacy to overcome possible feelings of hopelessness, powerlessness, loss of control, or fear associated with the diffuse threat of managed care. Through interactive learning participants come to recognize their membership in a community, where actors with different goals are dependent upon each other to make the system function effectively. Finally, the MCE/SP program established credibility from the start by presenting the strengths and weaknesses of the training so that participants could help improve it.

EMPOWERMENT THROUGH EVALUATION

MCE/SP labored intensively to assure that the program was accountable to administrators, internal consumers, patients, and other stakeholders. It built in numerous evaluation opportunities to help staff and participants reflect critically on the consequences of their action or praxis. The empowerment evaluation approach strives to provide asymmetrical, nonpaternalistic relationships by ensuring that the educational program reflects a learning *with* participants about the participants' work world. This commitment translated into a self-corrective *process evaluation* as an integral part of the implementation of the large-scale event technology. Thus after each training session, MCE/SP staff and internal facilitators meet to discuss new learning gained from carrying out an event; receive timely feedback regarding the usefulness of components of the particular educational module and efficacy of training materials; and document suggestions for program improvements. These debriefing sessions served to inform MCE/SP of what new material was needed; the cultural competence and acceptability of methods and components used; the performance of staff; and the feasibility of data collection.

More formal evaluation methods also were used: pre- and posttest of participants to measure attitude change after the intervention; and Likert-type scale survey questionnaires mailed to managed care coordinators and internal facilitators* at the conclusion of all educational sessions. The results of our evaluations are reported in detail, given the importance of evaluation as part of the empowerment solution and relevance for understanding the needs of diverse stakeholders.

---

*Managed care coordinators/facilitators co-led the educational modules throughout the six month intervention period. As trainers and representatives of front line and administrative titles, their evaluation results are instructive for future educational efforts.

Analysis of Key Evaluation Questions

This section summarizes findings from the post-session evaluation questionnaires submitted by attendees at sessions conducted from January 11 through June 30, 1994. Attendees were asked to fill out a questionnaire at the conclusion of the session. Ninety-three percent of attendees complied with this request. This report only includes results of the analysis for three key questions asked of the respondents. Responses were on a scale from A through E. These are:

1) Given what you knew about managed care in general, how would you rate the educational value of the training session?
2) Given what you knew prior to the session on the role of your job function in managed care, how would you rate the educational value of the training session?
3) Given that the entire training time consisted of one day (or one half-day for certain groups), how would you rate the overall value of the training experience?

Out of a total of 2,052 participants 1,918 (93%) responded to the questionnaire. Respondents by audience type were as follows: clerks (614), nurses (324), patient support staff (210), finance staff (309), allied health care staff (133), physicians and physician assistants (74), nurse practitioners/midwives (34), pharmacy staff (78), public relations staff and volunteers (24), risk management/QA/UR and credentialing staff (69), and directors (49).

Criteria for success of the education effort were that at least 80% of those responding to the particular question give a rating of either "I learned a great deal" or "I learned a moderate amount of information"; and at least 80% of those responding to the third question give a rating of at least "somewhat valuable." These criteria were met for all groups save physicians and allied health care staff/direct patient care staff (counselors, psychologists, social workers, and therapists). These audiences met the criteria in part. Nurse practitioners/midwives, however, did not meet any of the criteria.

Over 90% of all audiences except nurse practitioners/midwives rated the educational effort to be at least somewhat valuable on an overall basis. Four different audiences had 100% of respondents rating the overall sessions positively and 10 of the 11 groups gave 93% or more positive ratings. Over 80% of 8 of the 11 audiences indicated that they learned a great deal or a moderate amount. At least 74% of all but nurse practitioners/midwives rated the general educational value as positive. Eighty percent or more of 8 of the 10 audiences for which data was analyzed (allied health data was not calculated because the question was worded erroneously on the questionnaire) rated the educational value of the experience with respect to their specific role in managed care as positive. Only allied health and nurse practitioners/midwives showed less than 73% of positive responses on the item regarding the educational value for their specific roles.

When the responses for all attendees were combined for the first two questions, 90% of the total attendees rated the sessions as having a great deal of or moderate education value when considering managed care in general or their specific roles in managed care.

A summary of the responses for the question concerning the overall value of the educational experience indicates that 90% of the respondents rated the session as valuable or "valuable considering the time allowed." Some 98% of the total respondents regarded the session as at least somewhat valuable. Even when a weighted proportion is utilized, 94% of the respondents rated the sessions as at least somewhat valuable.

The results support the need for more audience-specific patient-care focused education. The value of these sessions has been demonstrated for a variety of HHC personnel including physicians, nurses, clerks, finance/MIS staff, patient support staff, pharmacy staff, public relations staff (including CABs and volunteers), and risk management/quality assurance/utilization review/credentialing staff. Respondents indicate that there is substantial learning both with regard to managed care in general and with reference to their job functions in relation to managed care.

The disaffection of the nurse practitioners may stem from the fact that HHC has not given them salary enhancements or recognized them as primary care practitioners in managed care at HHC even though they are eligible under state guidelines and despite the fact that HHC physician assistants (PAs) have been given this opportunity. This is a thorny issue because of the lesser educational experiences and credentials of PAs and because HHC has the authority to decide who will receive salary enhancements. Moreover, there is some indication that a substantial minority of the nurse practitioners/midwives may already have mastered much of the material presented. In this regard it is important to note that few respondents from any audience other than nurse practitioners/midwives indicated that this experience was in any way redundant of other training in which they participated. Directors and physicians may have had more knowledge going in than other groups so that the sessions, being half day, were too basic. Results from the nurse practitioners

and directors, as well as those attendees of the public relations modules must be reviewed with caution because of the small number of
respondents (34, 49, and 24, respectively).

Analysis of Facilitator's Questionnaires

Questionnaires were distributed to 50 managed care coordinators
and facilitators who along with Managed Care Education and Special Projects staff conducted the educational sessions throughout the
year. Twenty-six responses were received including responses from
18 facilitators and 8 other respondents for a total response rate of
52%. Facilitators responding included those who assisted in 10 of
the 11 types of modules that were conducted.

All respondents indicated that they felt themselves to be appropriately selected to facilitate the module or modules that they had
been assigned.

Regarding the question concerning the degree of comfort they felt
in carrying out the role of facilitator, 83% percent of the respondents
felt either very comfortable or comfortable about carrying out their
role as facilitator. Only two persons provided comments regarding
what it would take to increase comfort. One said, "time and practice"
and the other "if able to use role playing as was shown in the video."

The distribution of responses regarding the extent to which the
training was felt to be responsive to audience needs as rated by all
respondents was as follows: 65% of the respondents felt that the
training was responsive to audience needs to a great extent. However, over one-third of the respondents felt that the training is responsive only to some extent. Four of the six facilitators who
responded with "some extent" were facilitators for half-day modules
with one of the others not specifying which module he facilitated.
The majority of those responding "great extent" or "fairly great extent" were facilitators for full-day modules (although more than half
of those responding "great extent" were half-day facilitators). Again,
the differences by module type or length suggest a greater amount of
learning among lower level workers as compared to higher level
staff due to past knowledge of managed care being greater among
higher level staff.

The question regarding the type of education needed to help audiences successfully carry out their managed care roles as rated by facilitators and all respondents revealed that the most frequent option
selected was that of "More problem solving opportunities such as
case scenarios." Seventy-four percent of all respondents felt that
there should be more training in that area. Approximately two-thirds
of respondents felt that there should be "Follow-up to be sure that

the training is understood and mastered," and nearly half of the respondents felt that there should be "More training on specific roles."

Respondents were asked to rate each segment of the training as to
whether the particular component had "special merit," did not have
special merit but should be "retained," should be "changed" or
should be "eliminated."

At least 75% of the respondents felt that each segment either had
special merit or should be retained. Ratings for *Table Introductions*
were 100 percent. Table Introductions is the very first participative
activity each attendee engages in at the start of each workshop. Participants introduce themselves to each other by identifying name,
title, work location, past participation in large group events, and
what they expect to get out of the session. They select their own
recorders, presenters, and monitors who report to the whole group
on their table's commonalities, differences, and expected outcomes.
Facilitators note the audiences's diversity and commit to meeting
each participant's expectations before the session is over. A *Ques-
tion/Answer* panel that addressed urgent unanswered questions on
how managed care works received 94 to 95%. Taking special merit
ratings alone, the highest proportion of responses were for Table Introductions (86%) and the New Flow Process (82%). New Flow
Process refers to a 60 to 90-minute interactive learning segment presented to all audiences that reinforces understanding of Medicaid
Managed Care through participants role-playing the role of patient,
HMO representative, PCP, nurse, patient educator, specialist, and
clerk. Facilitators take the actors and larger audience through a new
"patient flow" process involving initial access into HHC's Managed
Care System, HMO Medicaid Managed Care Services, Primary Care
Clinic, Emergency Department triage, and patient education, inpatient area, and specialty clinics. Throughout, the "patient," other
actors, and the audience are provided details about enrollment
process/enrollee rights; disenrollment/grievance process; covered
services/noncovered services; authorization/notification procedures;
contractual issues/compliance; and cost-quality concerns. A core
component of the new flow activity is to provide to all participants,
a structural view of how patients have been taught dependency
upon emergency rooms (ER). Rather than solely ascribing inappropriate use of the ER to patient personality or cultural characteristics,
the activity highlights how infrastructure deficits, ethnocentric biases, and medical economic emphasis on specialty care has led to
institutional/provider and societal preference for crisis/catastrophic
medicine oriented delivery systems rather than preventive primary
care. The activity also provides participants with some basic information about national debates on rationalized care over a lifetime

versus "resurrection medicine," where heroic efforts and health expenditures occur at the initial and terminal stages of life.

The distribution of responses regarding the value of the training manuals/handouts (Learning Activities Manual, Introduction to Managed Care/Medicaid Managed Care Manual, Leader's Guide, and Information on the Metropolitan Health Plan) for facilitators and the distribution of responses regarding the value of these materials for the intended audience were: respondents generally felt the materials to be valuable for themselves. Seventy-five percent of the respondents felt the Learning Activities* Manual to be very valuable to the facilitators. Ninety-four percent of the respondents felt the Introduction to Managed Care[†] to be valuable or very valuable. Eighty-three percent rated the Leader's Guide and the information about the Metropolitan Health Plan as valuable or very valuable.

In terms of value to the audiences, well over 90% of the respondents rated the Learning Manual as valuable or very valuable; and approximately 85% rated the Introduction Manual and Metropolitan Health Plan information at that level.

Comments were solicited from the respondents regarding suggestions for additional handouts, information, and other comments. Materials suggested included a handout on the "new flow" process, more materials about sensitivity in relating to people in HHC's multicultural setting or on diversity, a separate sheet or card with specifics about the role of the target audience, and information on National Health Care Reform recommendations. It is instructive to note some of the comments from facilitators who worked with audiences consisting of health practitioners that have more direct patient care contact and responsibilities: present more practice applications and more information about Metropolitan Health Plan, and develop a program report or newsletter that addresses day-to-day questions.[‡]

---

*The Learning Activities Manual is an activity workbook that assists participants in following the design and structure of the educational session.

[†]The Introduction to Managed Care/Medicaid Managed Care Manual familiarizes participants with the New York State Managed Care Policy and Procedure Manual in a user-friendly format that also contains HHC specific information and presents a "customer centered" services approach (NYCHHC, 1994c, 1993a).

[‡]In September 1994, MCE/SP published "Managed Care Made Easy," answering 120 actual questions posed by HHC employees in educational sessions from January to June 1994. Answers are organized into the categories of concern expressed by managers, providers, and health care and support staff (NYCHHC, 1994b).

IMPLICATIONS FOR HHC/SAFETY NET PROVIDERS

A total of 3,350 persons attended educational or orientation sessions held by Managed Care Education and Special Projects. In addition to MCE/SP directed sessions, HHC facilities also conducted their own training in managed care, frequently including MCE/SP staff as advisors or as presenters. In total, training sessions reached well over 10,000 individuals.

As previously stated, MCE/SP offered a series of educational events from January 11, 1994, through June 30, 1994. A total of 57 events occurred with a total of 2,052 HHC staff members and volunteers participating. MCE/SP educated 623 clerks in ten full-day sessions; 335 RNs/LPNs and nursing aides in nine half-day sessions; 32 nurse midwife/practitioners in one half-day session; 83 physicians and physician assistants in seven half-day sessions; 80 risk management/quality assurance staff in three full-day sessions; 230 patient support staff in six half-day sessions; 144 allied health care staff in five half-day sessions; 29 public relations staff (including community advisory board members, volunteers and long-term care facility administrators) in two half-day sessions; 84 pharmacy staff in four full-day sessions; and 54 directors in three half-day sessions.

A total of 57 events have also been conducted by HHC facilities in addition to MCE/SP directed sessions. The importance to HHC of evaluating the educational empowerment initiative is that it helped us to identify the barriers and challenges faced by implementation of a managed care system if it is to be responsive. It enhanced our capabilities to identify possible solutions with the potential of adoption and ownership by diverse populations. Evaluation also has implications for other safety net providers who are interested in the generalizability of this health care reform intervention to their settings. Evaluating these internal marketing events clearly indicates the value of the activities for almost every audience reached. However, the approach has had some deficits: limiting the marketing methodology to the conduct of training sessions in general and large-scale events in particular; lack of coordination between HHC's Central Office and facility efforts; Central Office's bureaucratic controls and limited response to the problem of having large numbers of staff absent from important work functions. These limitations arose in the context of an administrative relationship between Central Office and the facilities that emphasized oversight and monitoring instead of support.

Experience in providing managed care education to all levels of HHC employees highlighted the value of training staff to understand their job functions under the new model of care. Pretraining evaluation results indicate major knowledge gaps among most staff. Posttraining results indicate that the training provided is of definite value. It is clear that intervention is required on a facility basis to assure that managed care is implemented in a manner that will maximize the benefit to HHC and its external customer base.

The experience also clearly demonstrated the importance of internal marketing. This type of marketing encompasses general information about managed care and the roles and specific activities necessary for staff to deliver managed care. The orientation that managed care education provides regarding the concept of managed care, its implications for revenue protection, strategies to maximize customer satisfaction, and the impact of managed care on different role functions should be continued.

To successfully continue, education should adopt a more flexible approach. That is, while the current stress on large-scale events (LSEs) enables reaching a large number of people in a short time, it has generated resistance. First, it is difficult to commit large numbers of key direct patient care staff—particularly physicians and, at times, nurses to educational sessions; second, it has been problematic for staff to travel long distances from their facilities for training. The delivery of training should be changed to accommodate these concerns by modifying the use of LSE technology to conduct training and by providing training on a regional basis.

Throughout the LSEs, MCE/SP found that it is feasible to attract sufficient numbers of clerks, patient support staff and, to a slightly lesser extent, finance staff to one meeting. However, it is not feasible to reach large numbers of physicians and nursing staff. Moreover, nursing staff and physicians require more than a half-day training. It is, therefore, recommended that physician training take place on a facility basis with physicians from D&TCs invited to their back-up hospitals.

Nursing orientation should also be conducted on a regional network-wide basis so that travel is minimized. Training clerks, patient support staff, and finance staff should continue as LSEs on a regional network-wide (rather than HHC-wide) basis. Finally, executive directors, training directors, and managed care coordinators should be queried regarding the content and future scheduling of LSEs for other staff (i.e., allied health and pharmacy staff).

Thus, instead of limiting the Central Office training approach to LSEs, education will vary according to the needs and reality of the audience (e.g., small group or seminar format). Moving toward a facility-network wide approach will also enable better coordination of sessions with training offered by the facilities which will reduce redundancy and maximize the value of training for the facility.

The impact of Medicaid Managed Care on HHC has at least two distinct dimensions—the impact on revenue and the impact on service utilization. The impact on revenue is the purview of finance. The impact on service utilization covers such areas as enrollment status, utilization rates of the emergency department and other services, waiting time, number of disenrollments, reason for disenrollments, number and nature of grievances, and patient satisfaction indicators. Monthly measurement of the status of the above factors and the degree to which managed care is being delivered according to state mandates are also important in determining the success of the program. Thus, recommendations for some of the areas which should be measured in the future include the extent to which:

- teamwork is practiced, with respect to service providers available, to serve enrollees in a coordinated fashion;
- care for each patient emphasizes case management;
- HMO and facility clerical staff communicate information concerning patient care, including authorizations and notifications;
- nonurgent emergency department patients are scheduled for physician visits on a timely basis;
- health educators are utilized to educate patients who inappropriately access services on how to correctly access the system;
- all staff understand the need for patient-centered services and act accordingly;
- all staff understand how to access all essential facility services so that they can correctly advise patients and visitors;
- referrals to specialty clinics are appropriate and are properly authorized by PCP and HMO; and
- specialty services are coordinated with the PCP.

SOCIAL MARKETING AND BEHAVIORAL HEALTH SYSTEMS

The preferred means of bringing about policy and organizational changes, given current movement away from traditional bureaucratic leadership in healthcare, is to advocate on behalf of managed care, educate staff to bring about action to implement managed care, and encourage key staff at facilities to assume greater control over the entire process (Green & Kreuter, 1991). A social marketing model built around the "health beliefs model" will be more effective in producing desired behavior around managed care. The model suggests that the message should be verbally and visually designed to convince the intended target groups that:

1) managed care will likely affect them;
2) it will have serious consequences when it does; and
3) the recommended behavior/action will reduce their susceptibility to severe financial consequences.

The approach must admit the shortcomings of the safety net's integrated care infrastructure and attempt to correct them. It involves a thorough analysis of the competition's strengths and weaknesses as well as the safety net's own managed care programs, products, and services. Among the factors that must be examined are the patients' perception of the convenience, effectiveness, and prestige of the safety net's managed care system as compared to competitors (Breckon, Harvey, & Lancaster, 1989).*

An internal social marketing approach recognizes that evaluation data becomes political and marketing data in the world of competitive Medicaid products (Green & Kreuter, 1991). An internal social marketing, community behavioral education approach differs from and complements traditional public affairs, marketing, communication, and outreach, and the facilities' individual related efforts. A combination of interventions at multiple levels is necessary to reach the varied constituents served by the safety net (Green & Kreuter, 1991).

The net's internal constituents include the board of directors, employees, medical staff members, volunteers, patients, community advisory board members, and friends of the facilities. MCE/SP trained facilitators identified as popular peer leaders from this internal constituency serve as behavior change endorsers who could contribute to a "multiplier effect." By doing so MCE/SP created the diffusion of innovation[†] effect necessary to promote rapid change. Hence, the task of future community health behavioral education is

---

*Thus, the patients' perceptions bring us back to the policy and planning issues of quality of care, ease of access, reasonable cost, freedom of choice, geographic location, personalized attention, medical outcomes, and whether customer service delivery is viewed as equal to private payer service.

†Diffusion of innovation theory posits that innovations are often initiated by a small segment of opinion leaders in a community. Once visibly modelled and accepted by such leaders, innovations then diffuse through a community, influencing others. Additionally, by focusing on frontline staff/health care providers who traditionally have counseled patients on what types of health services they need, patients are better informed and providers/staff appreciate their responsibility to teach patients health care access skills they were not taught under the old system of care.

to provide both the general environment and institutional support for managed care through policies, marketing, research, and management services to strengthen organizational readiness for further managed care product differentiation. Facility-based community health psychologists can collaborate and cooperate with the aforementioned entities in promoting the managed care message in internal newsletters, institutional brochures, annual reports, patient information booklets, advertising, and health education. Locating a community health behavioral education unit with a social marketing focus within each safety net facility would enable them to ethically attract new providers, to retain qualified health personnel and administrators, and to stay current in managed care service delivery (Snook, 1992).

Since the facilities should be primarily responsible for marketing on a facility, network wide, or regional basis, community health psychologists can act as internal senior management consultants to the executive directors (ED) and make recommendations as needed, including revitalizing coordination or collaboration among multiple facilities when similar problems are uncovered. Consultants can focus on making strategic planning one of the day-to-day activities of top managers by their incorporation of more long-range thinking and alternative goal setting to meet forecasted conditions. Community health psychologists can bridge the internal and external marketing needs of the safety net by continuing to maintain a common orientation in further educating employees at the facilities and sales/marketing representatives of the net's HMOs. Specifically, psychologists can utilize and modify the marketing, facilitation and presentation skills, cross-cultural communication and customer service orientation described in these pages (NYCHHC, 1994a, 1994d).

Community health psychology strategic planning helps physicians and other health services providers understand the decision processes and information that senior management and nonclinical staff use to assess quality outcomes, e.g., measuring and improving patient waiting and billing time; measuring and improving patients' and other external customers' satisfaction (Appel & Dunn, 1993). Community health organizational empowerment fundamentally rests on the belief that staff can empower themselves, reframe their perceptions of how to treat patients, enhance the implementation of the managed care model, and change their work environment. In carrying out its organizational development activities, community health behavioral education requires that changes recommended are feasible for the facility and workers affected, and that the workers who implement the changes recognize the benefits of such changes for their communities, worksites, and their own effective functioning.

CONCLUSION

It must be emphasized that managed care does not cure the symptoms of the U.S. health care system, rather it is a development that along with other trends makes it imperative for public/safety net agencies to position themselves as competitive health care providers of choice (Velez & Moshipur, 1993). The empowerment solution offered here is an extension of the basic premise of a community health psychology approach that seeks to empower communities of diversity to respond proactively to changes that can negatively impact on their quality of life. Communities of diversity refers both to those communities of consumers and of providers who have come together to collaborate on improving health for all while recognizing the difference of each.

In this regard, the sociopolitical environment that made our interventions possible at HHC occurred during a period of diversity, empowerment, and change within New York City government engendered by the election of David Dinkins, New York's first African American mayor. Significantly, he recruited and appointed commissioners and administrators of color to make city government more responsive to its majority minority populace. They sought to enhance the participation of citizens of color in the planning and implementation of health and human services, thus the HHC presidents appointed under his administration differed from past appointees in being persons of color *and* appreciative of psychology's role in service delivery and systems development. Thus this author and three other clinical-community psychologists emerged as key players in the restructuring of HHC into a community-oriented managed care system. Our roles as psychologist-administrators of color made a difference in our emphasis on empowerment of communities of diversity as a process and product. As professionals of color, we also encountered barriers related to not being part of the Caucasian network of "permanent government" and bureaucrats which historically has controlled municipal affairs. Both the acceptance and rejection of our diversity have marked our careers and personal lives, making us ever more committed to empowering solutions.

On a more individual level, my role as administrator, psychologist, consumer advocate, empowerment activist, and person of color, has led to many struggles to avoid being an apologist for the system, a proponent of managed care as a panacea, or of being blind to critiques of managed care, from within and outside of organized psychology. Indeed, there are many dangers in any gatekeeper system where profits are the primary concern. Diverse populations, psychologists serving their needs, and all of us are at risk of being un-derserved when necessary quality clinical services are not provided in a timely manner. Empowering patient-focused, consumer-oriented, community-informed, and culturally competent managed care systems cannot focus on shutting doors to care, rather they should create and facilitate access to pathways to appropriate care. Community health psychology, through social marketing, can blend the business wisdom of an educated consumer being the best cus-tomer with the social promise of knowledge being power to fashion healthy policy in the health business.

COMMENTARY

Tessie Guillermo

Community health institutions serving indigent, at-risk, communities of color throughout the country are struggling to prevail in the new world of health delivery known as managed care. Among the major threats is the institutions' ability to gain a competitive advantage over private sector competitors, particularly as Medicaid populations are now seen as a lucrative market segment for such competitors. Strategies employed are sometimes reactive, and often do not address adequately both the internal and external pressures that are brought to bear in assuring that the safety net of services are maintained over the long term.

Certain elements characteristic of organizations that successfully serve communities of color in an integrated service are required: 1) a solid database—scientific, empirical, statistical—with which to assess the communities' needs and the institution's impact on its target population; 2) strong ties to indigenous community institutions and a working knowledge of community social and cultural norms, which can make a health system more responsive and successful in meeting needs and create mutual respect and support between community and health providers; 3) involvement of communities of color in planning, implementation, and governance which requires advocacy, political activism, and policy competence on the part of providers and counterparts in the community; 4) consistent feedback mechanisms which assure that the health system will be responsive and dynamic with regard to the changing demographics and conditions of its community; ensure use of culturally competent survey and feedback mechanisms, and include data elements that allow for accurate identification of who is represented in the evaluation process; 5) effective case management which recognizes that the needs of communities of color are linked and require support services; and assures that services are provided in an appropriate community- or family-centered context; and 6) proactive outreach and education to the community which increases sensitivity to the conditions that surround the health system and its neighboring communities; and assists the constituents in overcoming their fears and dislike of the health care delivery system.

The experience in serving communities of color that the New York City Health and Hospitals Corporation (HHC) has, can put them at great advantage over their private sector competitors, if evaluated appropriately and disseminated throughout its newly empowered staff and restructured system. The approach described by Dr. De La

Cancela facilitates the integration of the above elements, and in fact, mirrors many of them as it focuses on alleviating the internal pressures of systems change.

Conventional wisdom relegates managed care to a simple matter of economics. Those who are tempted to maintain their criticism of managed care at this level will be left behind. By fully embracing integrated health systems (i.e., managed care in the ideal), safety net providers can assure they will be around in the long run to provide the quality care that at-risk populations and communities of color need. The marketing of managed care, whether to internal or external stakeholders, benefits greatly from an approach such as that employed by Dr. De La Cancela, whose ultimate goal is empowerment of all affected groups.

7

Cultural Diversity and Health Care Planning for Culturally Competent Services: A Community-Based Approach

Jean Lau Chin

OVERVIEW OF THE PROBLEM: CHANGE FROM THE OUTSIDE

As the population of the United States becomes increasingly diverse, health care planning must become culturally competent to meet the needs of diverse segments of the population. The concept of cultural competence is defined by Cross et al. in the monograph "Towards a Culturally Competent System of Care" (Cross, Bazron, Dennis, & Issacs, 1989), as a set of congruent behaviors, attitudes, and policies that come together in a system, agency, or amongst professionals and enables that system, agency, or those professionals to work effectively in cross-cultural situations. . . . A culturally competent system of care acknowledges and incorporates—at all levels—the importance of culture, the assessment of cross-cultural relations, vigilance toward the dynamics that result from cultural differences, the expansion of cultural knowledge, and the adaptation of services to meet culturally-unique needs.

This concept provides for the definition of cultural sensitivity at its broadest level. Too often, cultural sensitivity in human services implies a rather narrow view of examining only the culture of the client, i.e., the set of behaviors practiced by a client without looking at the system(s) and contexts in which services are provided. This concept applies to all aspects of a system of care, training, service delivery, and research. While initially developed for community mental health settings, it is also applicable to community-based organizations, community health centers, hospitals, public agencies, health maintenance organizations, and teaching institutions.

Although a move to cultural competence reflects a significant conceptual shift, its implementation within our health service delivery systems is still a far cry from success. Communities of color continue to face dilemmas in funding priorities and barriers in receiving culturally competent care. There are double binds that exist in the macro health care system. As cost containment measures drive the United States toward health reform, we need to ensure that any new system of care does not create new barriers or perpetuate old ones which have precluded communities of color from access to a culturally competent system of care.

SOCIOCULTURAL BARRIERS: A CASE EXAMPLE

Communities of color have historically faced sociocultural barriers in accessing health care services within the macro system of care: poverty, racism, unemployment, lack of insurance, language barriers, and cultural alienation are but some of them. Elimination of these barriers has been paramount to South Cove Community Health Center since its inception in 1972 when it was founded by a group of community activists within Boston's Chinatown. The primary source of health care for non-English speaking Chinese immigrants in the community was episodic care from the emergency room at the nearby medical center located within the neighborhood. The ability of providers to speak the language of the clients and to understand their culture was minimal. South Cove was founded to provide affordable and accessible primary care to low income, non-English speaking Asian immigrants and refugees. Its community board of directors was composed largely of Asian Americans who identified with, worked or live in the community, many of whom were second generation, whose parents or immediate families faced barriers to care (Chang & Tang, 1977; Issacs & Benjamin, 1991).

Crucial to the development of the health center was the vision of its founders, who recognized the importance of a center located in the community. Furthermore, they recognized the importance of service delivery by bilingual/bicultural providers, using a model of care sensitive to cultural values and practices.

The social context was also crucial. The emergence of second generation Chinese American immigrants able to speak and negotiate with mainstream institutions was key. Community organizations in

Chinatown were still in their infancy. Most of the community agencies were "multiservice" in nature, responding to the people who came for help, indiscriminate of professional specialties. The Chinese immigrants just needed someone to negotiate the Western system for them.

Also important as a context was the ongoing community mental health movement in the country. Asian social workers were organizing nationwide in response to the civil rights movement of the 1960s. The National Institute of Mental Health hosted a conference in 1972 in which 300 Asians came from across the nation seeking services for underserved segments of their communities. The Boston contingent came back, energized and ready to advocate locally for services to the Asian community. Many were the founders of the present agencies in Boston's Chinatown.

Now, more than 20 years later, barriers in accessing health care continue to exist. They are financial: 56% of Asians in Chinatown are uninsured. They are cultural and linguistic: many immigrants and refugees are unfamiliar with Western medicine, culture, and health practice; many speak limited English. In addition, these barriers have been evident within the macro system as we have advocated to bring affordable health care to the community.

In the 1990s, South Cove responded to the diversity within the community of Asians from China, Hong Kong, Taiwan, Vietnam, Cambodia, Malaysia, Thailand, Singapore, and the Philippines. We provide a comprehensive range of primary and preventive care services to over 10,000 clients a year. Eighty percent of our staff of 150 speak at least one Asian dialect with a capacity for over 10 different Asian languages/dialects in addition to English. The majority of our clients are now Chinese, Vietnamese, and Cambodian immigrants and refugees who are primarily non-English speaking, low income, and often uninsured. Our comprehensive range of services, conceived of as "one-stop shopping," includes significant community outreach and health education. Essential to our service delivery is the strength of our community-based networks.

Our clients now come from over 30 different towns/neighborhoods in greater Boston reflecting our regional focus. Given the limited availability of affordable housing, many Asians have moved or settled outside the immediate neighborhood while continuing to identify with and use Chinatown for its services. Still, the macro system often does not have regulations or the flexibility to recognize our population focus in its funding priorities. We are still viewed as an exception which threatens the integrity of a mainstream system unable to meet the needs of the Asian community. Agencies recruit our bilingual staff as we compete for scarce human resources targeting the Asian community. Agencies use our translated materials and rely on our staff for consultation and interpreter support. Yet, few of their resources support the infrastructure needed to support our costs. While the Asian population has tripled over the past decade, there are often no additional resources from local and state funders for the larger number of underserved Asians because their numbers are still considered too small. The absence of data fails to document their need. The very success of our model often makes us ineligible for resources directed at new initiatives for cultural competence and capacity building.

The urgency of cost containment, spread of managed care, and privatization driving the movement for reform have shifted our focus. Primary care and community health centers are now in a competitive market. Whereas the underserved and uninsured, and disenfranchised people of color were once persona non grata in the private sector, we now find for-profits competing for our patients. In response to these emerging contexts, South Cove began to establish itself as a regional primary and preventive care center for Asians in greater Boston. We have expanded our scope to meet the needs of the growing Asian population through multiple sites in neighborhoods where high concentrations of Asians reside.

However, sociocultural barriers continue to exist. For poor and low-income communities of color who face language, cultural, and financial barriers to care, the ability to provide quality health care services is insufficient to guarantee access to care. Linguistically appropriate services at all points of patient contact which is not limited to interpreter support are needed to ensure a patient-oriented approach to quality care. Staff who are knowledgeable about the client's culture and part of the community are key to designing a practice which is relevant to the health needs of the community. Community outreach, which includes health education and information dissemination in the primary language of the clients, is essential to bring people into care. Case management services are needed to facilitate the movement of clients through a system which is often unfamiliar and alien to their cultural values, health beliefs, and established habits.

While such services are essential to promote access to care, they are not reimbursable through third party insurance. Advocacy has been essential to obtain the resources necessary to support this comprehensive and community-based system of care. We have long provided "one stop shopping" as clients sought us out for multiple services well beyond traditional definitions of medical care, i.e., escort services, bill translation, interpreter support, assistance in filling out applications, and letter writing. We targeted health risks such as hepatitis B, thalassemia, diabetes, and tuberculosis before they were viewed as larger public health threats because they were prevalent in the Asian community.

PRINCIPLES OF COMMUNITY-BASED CARE

Our system of care would be meaningless without the principles underlying their significance. First, the principle of community-based services is inherent to our role as a community health center. Our clients know and trust us, and often use our staff as gatekeepers for those who seek entry to the community, i.e., researchers and trainees. We have our finger on the pulse of the community, and therefore, are the first to anticipate and know those issues impacting the health of our community. We are familiar, first hand, with the clinical practices which will succeed or fail in the community because of the feedback provided to us through formal and informal community networks.

Second, the principle of cultural competence is key to quality of care. As the United States population has become increasingly diverse, the need for cultural sensitivity has shifted toward a need to become culturally competent. This principle prescribes that health care providers and systems of care should not only know, but also value and integrate cultural beliefs, practices, and knowledge into health care delivery. At South Cove, we grappled with the fact that our patients use herbal medicine simultaneous with our prescription of Western medicine without devaluing its cultural importance or defining this practice as noncompliance. We attended to the changing population demographics as the Asian community in greater Boston became increasingly diverse with Chinese immigrants from many different countries speaking multiple dialects, and the rapid influx of Southeast Asian refugees. We struggled with the ethical responsibilities as community-based providers might meet clients seeking advice as they shopped and used community services themselves.

Lastly, the principle of linguistic appropriateness enables true rapport with the client. This is cited last because it is all too easy to confuse language as the first and only criterion for serving a linguistically different population. Moreover, removing barriers to care is too often reduced to the provision of interpreter support alone by nonmonitored and poorly trained interpreters.

COMMUNITY INFRASTRUCTURES

Important as are the principles underlying care, an infrastructure is needed to institutionalize a macro system of health care which opens its doors to all segments of the population. For years, South Cove focused on the services and principles necessary to remove sociocultural barriers to care. We played a strong advocacy role to ensure that the voices of underserved segments of the Asian community were heard. However, it is increasingly clear that this is insufficient if the macro system is unresponsive and culturally incompetent in addressing the needs of specific segments of the population. It means that systemic and institutionalized mechanisms must exist to promote and permit practices which differ from those in the "mainstream." It means that we must acknowledge the bias of existing frameworks which define and prescribe practices which may be inadequate for some segments of the population. It means a continued need to advocate on behalf of those voices in the community still to be heard. These are the barriers we have yet to overcome completely.

For example, South Cove has a "labor coach" model in which pregnant women are supported prior to and during their delivery. Through this relationship, interpreter support, case management services, continuity of care, and psychosocial support are provided. Yet, the services are not reimbursable; we often need to justify their necessity to funding sources who view them as a luxury. Some will ask, "Why don't their husbands support them?" without realizing that many husbands do not get paid leave time, do not speak English, do not know the health care system, and are working six days a week for 10 hours each day.

Part of the success of our approach is due to our provision of extensive community outreach and health education to inform the community about health risks and promote early entry into care. We translate and develop multilingual and culturally relevant materials to reach the non-English speaking Asian community. These efforts are time consuming, resource intensive, and require regular updating. Yet, our materials are often used by other health providers without acknowledgment or compensation for the infrastructure needed to sustain these activities.

As health care reform becomes equated with managed care, geography is increasingly used as the primary criterion in defining access to care. For community health agencies focusing on a specific ethnic population, new barriers are created which prevent us from serving our target population. Our clients choose to travel longer distances to access a comprehensive, bilingual/bicultural system of care; yet, service area and geographic boundaries have defined our services as out of bounds for those clients. We have also faced more cumbersome administrative work in multiple forms, contracts, and proposals because our clients overlap service areas with multiple jurisdictions.

Lastly, the system of care targeting a specific linguistic, ethnic population has often been viewed as temporary; that is, to exist only until our clients can speak English or the mainstream system can serve them. These are the challenges and sociocultural barriers still to be overcome. The U.S. macro health care system fails to support the infrastructures needed to serve ethnic specific populations. Systemic change is needed to promote cultural competence within a macro system which recognizes and allows, through its regulations and priorities, different and multiple options for low incidence populations whose needs may not fit a "mainstream" definition.

EVOLUTION AND DEVELOPMENT OF CULTURAL COMPETENCE

The cultural competence of a system needs to occur at all levels including: 1) policy/governance, 2) administrative, 3) practice/service, and 4) consumer/community. In examining the evolution and development of issues at each of these levels within South Cove's history, we can capture the developmental stages of this community based approach to health care planning and service delivery.

Policy/Governance

First, we revised our mission twice in response to the growing diversity of our population. From Chinese Health Center, our name was revised to South Cove Community Health Center. Our mission statement changed our single focus on the Chinese population to include Asians. Initially, the demand for our services resulted in increased requests for interpreter support at hospitals and other human service agencies. As this expanded even beyond health care services, often without reimbursement, our policy shifted toward one of not providing interpretation services because we prided ourselves on our bilingual/bicultural care. Our population grew increasingly diverse, and our clients now speak multiple Asian dialects. While 80% of our staff speak at least one Asian dialect, a bilingual provider may not always speak the dialect spoken by the client. As a result, we have once again modified this policy and developed a more complex system of multilingual support to our clients. The valuing of bilingual/bicultural skills through recruitment, operational procedures, and compensation packages empowers staff toward community-based and culturally competent values.

Administrative

At the administrative level, many decisions are guided by the emphasis on cultural competence. A priority is given to Asian bilingual physicians in our recruitment efforts. We expanded our strategies toward a national recruitment to increase the pool of candidates, and built on community networks to identify potential candidates. Asians are prominent at all levels of our administrative structure.

Day-to-day decisions such as holidays are made with attention to sensitivity to culture. Our personnel policy was revised to enable staff to take extended time off in recognition that many are themselves immigrants and refugees with families outside the United States; regular requests for extended leave time were often associated with the wish to spend time with families overseas.

As the demand for our services grew and we did not have the space and resources to see all who came, we made decisions to refer Asian clients able to speak some English to other health care providers given our priority to serve the large unmet needs of non-English–speaking Asians.

Practice/Service

Our clinical practices are modified by the health beliefs, practices, and values of our patients. This includes the modification of nutritional foods and units of measures consistent with an Asian diet as well as the modification of recommendations about prenatal care consistent with known practices among Chinese, Vietnamese, and Cambodian women.

Our services have always prioritized those health risks prevalent among the Asian population. The growth of our pediatric and obstetrical services was driven by the demand for our services. While herbal medicine and acupuncture derive from the Asian culture, it has not been integrated into our practice. This may have reflected the fact that herbalists and acupuncturists already practiced in the community. Our early attempts to address an unmet need by offering a culturally and clinically competent Western form of health care, and to avoid competition within the community, precluded our attempts to offer these services. Given the current integration of acupuncture in some substance abuse and HIV/AIDS treatment programs, we may begin to reevaluate this issue toward a more integrative approach.

With reform measures under discussion, we are reviewing our practices with an eye toward how managed care systems can be responsive to the needs of the Asian community.

Consumer/Community

As a community health center, South Cove has always been a part of the Asian community. We are located in Boston's Chinatown, and our staff are often themselves part of the community. In addition, we conduct focus groups regularly to assess feedback from the community on our services vis à vis community health needs. We are often informed about community issues through our participation in community activities.

The attention to cultural competence at all levels of our organization is a process that is ongoing and evaluative. Our ties with the community place a responsibility for us to advocate with and provide leadership for health care issues relevant to the Asian community.

THE DOUBLE BIND IN PLANNING

Mainstream vs. Ethnic Specific Services

While funding priorities have shown an increased awareness of and sensitivity to cultural diversity as a goal, health care planning often emphasizes a dichotomy between "mainstream" agencies and "ethnic-specific" agencies. Mainstream agencies are funded as "broad" in purpose even though they are increasingly deficient in providing the services needed by ethnic- and linguistic-specific populations. Many do not have the language capacity, cultural competence, or staffing patterns needed to serve linguistically diverse populations.

Mainstream agencies are often mandated to work with and serve ethnically diverse populations within their geographic areas. This often leads them to seek out "ethnic" agencies as cultural experts, or to offer themselves as consultants to these agencies in meeting their mandates. However, community empowering relationships or financial resources are generally not associated with these arrangements, leaving ethnic agencies bearing the burden of subsidizing the services of mainstream agencies.

While the need to communicate with clients in their primary language is clear, the mainstream emphasis is often on seeking translators rather than bilingual providers. Translation services are often viewed as ends in themselves rather than as transitional solutions. Consequently, professionals of color are often marginalized as second class citizens valued only for their ethnicity. Without financial resources or clinical decision making shared with ethnic agencies, duplication of services, higher costs, and administrative inefficiencies will occur.

Recruitment and Retention of Ethnic Staff

Mainstream agencies and institutions often claim difficulty in finding qualified ethnic staff. Nevertheless, their criteria for recruiting and utilizing professionals of color is often reduced to language alone. Mainstream agencies often do not seek out community networks for recruiting ethnic professionals into the field.

Ethnic professionals face the additional dilemma of being pigeonholed in having their expertise defined solely by their ability to speak a language other than English, or because of their ethnic identity. Consequently, ethnic professionals from communities of color face the dilemma of having their career paths narrowly defined by ethnicity rather than clinical competence.

Needs Assessment: How big is the problem?

The United States is a society fascinated by large numbers. We count everything. We compare everything. When it comes to communities of color, we are defined by our smaller numbers. Census tract data often used to document need and allocate resources are inadequate in capturing these needs. Asian Americans, for example, are often deemed too few to be counted, and are often omitted from national, state, and local datasets. When included, they are often listed as "Other" or lumped together in ways that mask their needs.

Despite health disparities, epidemiological data generally show that Asians do not have an easily identifiable health problem. The low prevalence of problems on key health indicators are often cited as evidence to justify the failure to allocate resources. Ignored are the different indicators relevant to health needs and disparities within the Asian community. As a result, low priority is given to allocating resources to Asians because their numbers do not fit the mainstream parameters of need. To be responsive to these communities, qualitative data via ethnographic methods is more useful. Interpretation of data needs to be viewed from the standpoint of community members. To ensure this, we need to be able to question the sanctity of traditional methods and recognize that communities of color can represent differing needs.

Difference vs. Norms

The emphasis on normative data forces communities of color to justify their existence compared to the mainstream. Immigrants are acculturated into Western culture. Communities of color are viewed as more or less than whites on a given trait. Communities of color practice alternative methods of healing. Non-English–speaking groups need "ethnic-specific" rather than "mainstream" services. Practices which must be adapted to meet the needs of specific communities are considered deviations from standard practice. These dichotomies presume that current health care practices should be universal, and culture is presumed to be a secondary variable. These dichotomies fail to acknowledge and promote options for communities with diverse needs who want different solutions.

CULTURALLY COMPETENT APPROACHES TO CHANGE: A COMMUNITY-BASED APPROACH

While health care planning needs to be responsive to cultural diversity and attain cultural competence, we need to move beyond paying lip service to the concept. We need to start by modifying those concepts that currently lead our service delivery system toward providing incompetent care. The impact of policy and funding priorities which define criteria irrelevant to the needs and realities of communities of color need to be mitigated. We need to provide incentives and mandates which influence culturally competent outcomes. Finally, we need to develop culturally competent models at all levels which are inclusive of all segments of the population, which are community based, and which promote comprehensiveness in providing continuity of care.

These elements need to be present in our service delivery systems, training curricula, research design, and evaluation criteria. Evaluation of cultural competence needs to occur throughout all levels of a system: policy/governance, administrative, practice/service, training, consumer/community.

Successful community-based approaches include the provision of extensive health education, community outreach, case management, interpreter support, and the availability of bilingual/bicultural providers. For example, South Cove began blood pressure screening and cholesterol screening through our health fairs long before the public health sector recognized and acknowledged its importance for Asian Americans. Our role as advocate serves to identify gaps in services where the macro system has been unresponsive. We knew that tuberculosis was epidemic in the Asian community long before it gained national attention as a public health risk. We developed special initiatives to target those health risks prevalent in the Asian community which were ignored in the mainstream. South Cove began screening, counseling, and outreach for thalassemia (a genetic blood disorder similar to anemia with a 14% carrier rate in the Asian population) long before people had even heard of the term. We began immunization of babies born to hepatitis B positive carrier mothers before universal immunization of Asian mothers was recommended by the Centers for Disease Control. Both these diseases have carrier rates of about 14% in the Asian population compared to less than 1% in the white population. Our recent study of diabetes shows a 10% prevalence in our population compared to a 4% prevalence in the white population. Substance abuse and AIDS have grown at alarming rates despite their low prevalence in the Asian population. Depression and suicide rates for Asian Americans exceed those for other groups when we look at specific age and ethnic groups, i.e., teenagers and older Chinese women.

CONCLUSION

In conclusion, health care planning must reflect the cultural diversity within our communities. The need to review our assumptions and values to promote a system of health care which addresses all segments of the population is essential. We must strive toward a system that is culturally competent. In this community-based approach, we face the double bind of being community providers on the outside looking in, yet a part of the community being served. We are both provider within the system, and advocate to change the system of which we are a part. Our community health psychology approach helps to identify essential elements of a culturally competent system in which we must:

- value diversity and accept differences;
- have the capacity for cultural self-assessment;
- be conscious of interacting dynamics of cultures;
- institutionalize the cultural beliefs and values of the community into our clinical practices;
- develop diverse solutions to meet different needs of our diverse communities; and
- implement the principles throughout all levels of a system, i.e., policy, administrative, practice, and community.

COMMENTARY

Herbert M. Joseph, Jr.

While the challenges posed by planning and implementing a cultur-ally competent health care system seem enormous and overwhelm-ing, the opportunities for unique and creative responses to these challenges probably represent the best hope for communities of color, in particular, to have access to and collaborate in designing health care systems relevant to their needs. The South Cove Community Health Center, a greater Boston area regional primary care health center, is a case in point, in that it seeks to provide comprehensive and culturally competent health care service to Asian populations.

As a general notion, the integration of the concept of cultural competence in the design of health care service systems could be characterized by a dynamic continuum of stages (see Cross, et al., 1989) which agencies and institutions may move through or remain stuck at as they seek to provide care to diverse populations. Many traditional models of health care delivery have not been designed to respond to the needs of the underserved and people of color at their inception. In some cases, the incorporation of cultural issues was never perceived to be relevant to their mission (cultural blindness), while in some others paternalism or ignorance (cultural incapacity) have been the dominant postures.

As a matter of equal and emerging concern has been the recent proliferation of health care groups, agencies, and organizations who have jumped on the "cultural diversity bandwagon," often in re-sponse to demands from funders, accrediting bodies, and, in some few cases, the communities they serve. It is important to recognize the effect that these "add on" cultural diversity efforts may have upon the larger system of care in community settings. First, these ef-forts are often designed from the "top down" rather than the "bot-tom up" or, preferably, in the horizontal, collaborative fashion, where members of the affected communities are partners in the planning process right from the start. Second, little attention is paid by the agency to assessing its own cultural competence, the belief being that it is sufficient to engage in one-sided learning of the his-tory, beliefs, and customs of "the other" rather than "ourselves in re-lation to the other." This is a fallacy which is all too common among newcomers to the area of cultural competence, who also see culture as static and monolithic rather than dynamic and characterized by diversity within a group diversity.

Third, the impact of the larger ecology, specifically the impact of racism and discrimination, poverty, and toxic environments, on the

*health, well-being and quality of life of communities can be mini-
mized by those seeking a "cultural" explanation for behavior. Finally, one is left with the impression that cultural diversity and
difference run the risk of being marginalized rather than being made
an integral part of the design of health care delivery systems. This is
exemplified by an agency with an ethnic-specific program aimed at
a particular group. While in some ways laudable, this type of program is often held captive by a number of internal and external
forces operating in or around the agency, including poor resource allocation (compared to other mainstream programs), little or no flexibility in contracting for services to meet the needs of the particular
population, and being a "special" program, resulting in agency (staff
and administrators) bearing little or no responsibility for serving the
population except through the particular program. What then arises
are issues of staff retention, burnout, and the impact of "ghettoiz-
ing" a program, likely increasing its sense of isolation and marginalization within the agency.*

*The South Cove Community Health Center model which this
chapter discusses may represent the hope and opportunity for the
delivery of agency-wide, planned, culturally competent, community-
based care to the natural diversity which exists within the Asian
community. The health center's beginning rested upon community
residents who had a vision of providing health care to non-English–speaking Asian immigrants and refugees from low-income
groups. This vision has continued while services have expanded. By
recognizing and valuing community collaboration in service design
and delivery, by being multiservice oriented, by being activist and
preventive in its approaches to care, and by taking the risk of assessing its own cultural competence as an agency, the South Cove
Center offers a prime example of a health care delivery system that
is moving along the continuum toward cultural proficiency (Cross, et
al, 1989).*

*All in all, some lessons can be abstracted from the South Cove's
culturally competent model. Some of these are:*

*1) The community (or communities) must be true, active, and equal
partners in the design and delivery of the health care system (s)
in their own communities. This should range from community
needs assessment, program design, evaluation, advocacy, and
program leadership and support through paid or volunteer roles.*

*2) Agencies must be open and willing to do some form of self-
assessment when it comes to the area of cultural competence (see
Cross, et al., 1989 for one model).*

3) *Systems of care should be integrated in such a way that communities can be served through "one-stop shopping" models.*

4) *Resources should be allocated fairly and in such a way as to allow for accountability as well as flexibility. This speaks to the need for solidly funded initiatives that will support pooled rather than categorical funding streams so as to maximize the resources available in communities, and encourage cross-collaboration and shared or regional program designs whenever possible.*

5) *Recruitment and retention of bilingual/bicultural staff (including training initiatives) should be considered a high priority in light of the shifting demographics which will put people of color in the United States increasingly in the majority. The impact of health providers who "speak the language" should not be underestimated.*

In sum, despite the challenges which cultural diversity poses to health care, there also exist enormous opportunities for health care administrators, funders, providers, and communities to work together to develop innovative and creative responses to the delivery of health care in culturally diverse communities. This should be one of the goals of community health psychology as we approach the twenty-first century.

8

Embracing People of Color: Implications for College Mental Health Services

Yvonne M. Jenkins

In the United States, much of what has determined access to quality health, mental health care, and health education has been associated with race, social class, and gender. Since health care systems have primarily been shaped by dominant culture perspectives and disempowering social inequities, people of color and the poor continue to be prevalent among underserved populations. This reality has important implications for community health psychology. Furthermore, it has important implications for collaboration between mental health services at senior level colleges and universities and mental health resources in the communities that surround them.

Colleges and universities are microcosms of the larger society. Even though the quality of counseling and mental health services for students tends to be more accessible and comprehensive than that typically offered to the general public, students of color at predominantly white universities are still too often shortchanged. In addition, the needs of mixed race, multicultural, immigrant, foreign national students, and others marginalized by difference are too often neglected by college mental health facilities. Because identity development (psychological and social), personality integration, personal and relational competence, and achievement are influenced by diversity and how it is responded to, college mental health services have an ethical responsibility to provide culturally competent care and training.

Even though significant milestones toward fairness, equity, and mutuality have been achieved through legislation, progressive education (i.e., diversity workshops, culturally competent curricula), and good will, oppressive mindsets and practices are still evident in some aspects of college mental health service delivery. Therefore, this chapter highlights challenges that increasingly diverse student populations pose to traditional college mental health services.

Although *valuing difference* is a familiar term within politically correct circles on campuses, many students of color are painfully aware of the difference in its use as rhetoric and the reality of their daily experiences. With this in mind, this chapter discusses some ways in which college mental health services can embrace diversity more effectively through providing culturally competent services and training. At a broader community level, it emphasizes the need for collaboration between college mental health administrators and practitioners, schools of medicine and public health, community health psychologists, teaching hospitals, community health and mental health facilities, and relevant research projects. Moreover, it recognizes that college mental health practitioners are potentially valuable resources for preventive health and mental health endeavors on campuses as well as in the community.

CHANGING TRENDS IN PSYCHOLOGICAL AND SOCIAL HEALTH

College populations hold much promise. Qualities like youth, vitality, resilience, creativity, and motivation for self-improvement have typically enabled this population to benefit enormously from counseling and psychotherapy. Yet, in recent years changes are evident in the complexity and severity of problems presented by students that seem to be influenced by multiple factors: more positive perceptions of helpseeking than in the past; acceptance of the disease model as an alternative to blaming the victim; increasingly complex societal problems and health issues; the changing structure of the family; the increasing population of first generation college students; technological advances that facilitate nearly instant communication while at times compromising human capacities for empathy, intimacy, interpersonal authenticity and mutuality, and frustration tolerance.

SOCIAL AMBIANCE

Each college and university has a distinct social ambiance. Not only does it impact on the overall development of students but it also influences the mindset and practices of surrounding communities. The social ambiance of an institution involves how that institution responds to diversity at every level of campus life. It involves everything from the most subtle nuances of daily life to the most visible expressions of acceptance and rejection.

The social ambiance for predominantly white colleges and universities is influenced by the nature of that institution's relationship with people of color from its inception. Answers to questions like the following may be useful for clarifying that relationship: When was the university founded? When were students of color first admitted? How enthusiastic has the university been about recruiting qualified students and staff of color? How many students from specific racial and ethnocultural groups have applied for admission and have been accepted during the past decade? Of those, what percentage graduated? What percentage dropped out or transferred to other institutions? Why? Is there any past or current documentation of the experiences of former students that pertains to race relations? If so, how did they describe their experiences? Have organized student protests related to diversity ever taken place on campus? If so, when and what motivated these protests? What public images does the institution have in relation to students of color? Do students of color feel valued or devalued on campus? Why? Are people of color generally viewed as affirmative action quota-fillers or as competent and deserving? What campus organizations are available to students of color on the basis of ethnocultural or racial identity? Are students of color adequately represented among elected or appointed officers of other student organizations? How involved are former students of color with alumni activities, particularly annual giving campaigns? What percentage of the faculty and administrators are people of color? What percentage of college counselors or mental health practitioners are people of color? How do these percentages compare with the number of students of color enrolled? Do students of color feel as though their needs are met adequately by campus counseling and mental health services?

The social ambiance of an institution of higher learning is vital to the sense of agency or empowerment felt by students. All people have ethnic and cultural origins that influence their ways of perceiving, responding to, and living in the world. Therefore, when the social ambiance of an institution embraces and celebrates diversity, the university community and society at large have much to gain.

WHO ARE STUDENTS OF COLOR?

Bowser, Arietta, and Jones (1993) remind us that the United States and its colleges and universities are still stratified by color. In this chapter, *students of color* refers to United States and international students of African, Asian, Latin-American, or Native American ancestries who study in the United States. As such, this is a very heterogeneous group from a myriad of ethnicities, cultures, and lifestyles. There is also considerable diversity of physical character- istics. Inasmuch as skin color is a prominent determinant of social identity in the United States, *students of color* is a highly political term in that it includes those for whom racism and oppression are most intractable.

It is expected that by the year 2000, more students of color than ever before will be attending colleges and universities in the United States. This has profound implications for college mental health ser- vices in regards to staffing and the need to examine guiding theoretical orientations, intervention, outreach strategies, advocacy, and training.

EMBRACING DIVERSITY

The process of embracing diversity involves a state of mind and a way of being. The cognitive dimension of this process involves movement toward increased social self-understanding and resolu- tion of personal barriers (e.g., prejudice, internalization of stereo- types) that block openness to difference. Embracing diversity also involves becoming more knowledgeable of both the local and global world communities as well as the growth evidenced by the unfold- ing of a more flexible and socially contextualized perspective of human relational development than traditional frameworks have en- compassed. The practice dimension of this process is active. It ini- tially involves clarifying and appreciating one's own social identity and openness to possibilities for mutually valued interaction with those who are different. As such, both subject and object are en- larged by this process just as both would be deprived of possibilities for growth and would suffer indignities if diversity was devalued.

Valuing Diversity on Campus

When diversity is valued, *all* students feel valued and connected to the university community. They feel understood, accepted, cared about, and supported. Confidence that their strengths are appreci- ated assures them that their presence matters. Students who feel val- ued share a sense of camaraderie with their peers. School pride, reflected by a personal sense of belonging, ownership, and interest in school-related endeavors is readily apparent. Discriminatory stan- dards of behavior and academic performance do not exist. Therefore, the presence of students of color on various campus locations does not automatically render them targets of suspicion by security, residence staff, or others in authority. Furthermore, students of color may comfortably sit together in dining halls or other places on campus without automatically being perceived as threatening or suspicious. When diversity is valued, *all* students can trust that their best interests are taken to heart by those in authority. Administrators, professors, and student personnel and supportive services are open to change (i.e., progressive ideas and new experiences). It is acknowledged that difference does indeed matter. Furthermore, the strengths of different lifestyles as well as the commonalties of human experiences are appreciated (Chin, De La Cancela, & Jenkins, 1993). A sense of mutual value exists between students, administrators, professors and other authority figures despite obvious power differentials. Students of color are not humiliated, ignored, or objectified through exoticism, fantasy, or tokenism. Course content reflects openness and a socially contextualized view of the world, and acknowledges the relationship between the current plight and history of disenfranchised groups in the United States. Affirmative language is used to refer to these groups rather than that which offends and perpetuates oppression. When diversity is valued, students are only held accountable for themselves rather than pressured to represent an entire reference group (e.g., race, gender, culture). Moreover, institutions that genuinely value diversity recognize the limitations of standardized admissions tests for accurate measurement of the skills and abilities of those whose backgrounds and social realities differ from traditional norm groups. In addition, there is an openness to including culturally competent supplemental measures.

Finally, when diversity is valued, it is visible in staffing and the student body. Optimal efforts are expended to find a successful model of "recruiting and training [qualified] people of color as students and faculty" and "to involve colleagues of color in shaping plans, goals, and agendas" for academic departments and health services (Bowser, Arietta, & Jones, 1993). All of this mobilizes hope and encourages the realization of dreams.

When Diversity Is Not Valued

When diversity is not valued, students tend to feel unworthy, marginalized, and estranged from the campus community. Feelings of alienation, isolation, and rejection are also common to their experience. Students of color who do not fit the stereotypes created by the dominant culture are considered anomalies, or exceptions to the rule since negative images of the reference group are prevalent. In addition, a student may feel undue pressure to represent an entire reference group, or to succeed in order to fulfill the hopes and dreams of loved ones and others who are deeply invested in his or her success or to disprove stereotypes about the abilities or moral character of the group. At times, this is at the cost of foregoing helpseeking or acknowledging vulnerability in any way. There are also instances when students of color feel the need to protect or not disappoint faculty of color; this causes considerable anxiety. In some instances, negative perceptions of difference are internalized and projected onto others, thereby perpetuating the cycle of oppression. This may result in self-hate as well as estrangement from one's own reference group. The pressure of intense scrutiny, discriminatory standards of accountability, and routine suspicion inevitably generates tension and insecurity. In other instances, what might appear on the outside to be a less vulnerable demeanor is evidenced by apathy, indifference, hostility, or aggression. Yet, what usually lies at the core are unfulfilled needs for acceptance, affirmation, and connection. Unfortunately, diversity is too often devalued. Thus, some students of color and other special populations are not adequately nurtured, supported, or mentored during critical years of psychosocial and career development.

What enables diversity to be valued? Diversity is valued through: (1) self-understanding, (2) development of a solid social and political identity, (3) cultural or multicultural education, (4) knowledge of how history and sociopolitical processes impact on different groups in the United States, and (5) relationships based on mutuality, empathy, and authenticity (Jenkins, De La Cancela, & Chin, 1993; Jordan, Kaplan, Miller, et al., 1991; Pinderhughes, 1989). In order to value diversity in others, one's own social identity must be clear and positive. Pride in one's own reference group and background (i.e., social, political, personal), and awareness of one's own internal experience of difference. To achieve a clear and positive social identity, perceptions, attitudes, and feelings about one's own identity must be owned, explored, and, if necessary, worked through. This process must be ongoing.

Barriers to valuing diversity must be eliminated. Active and authentic engagement in relationships with members of other reference groups over time influence accurate perceptions. With first-hand knowledge of different world views, lifestyles, and cultural practices, fantasy, stereotypes, and action that devalue diversity are less likely to persist. In addition, awareness of the impact of history and sociopolitical processes on particular groups is conducive to understanding their worldviews and the daily social realities encountered. Domination, marginalization, and exclusion are common to the backgrounds of people of color in the United States. Awareness of the impact of various sociopolitical processes on a specific group is also relevant to its accessibility to various resources, and how it is perceived and responded to both within the group and in the larger society. How diversity is responded to in counseling and psychotherapy is central to probabilities for healing and recovery.

The Centrality of the Relationship to Intervention with Pluralistic Populations

The relationship is central to treating pluralistic populations. Personal warmth, approachability, and genuineness are central to establishing the types of growth-fostering relationships with consumers associated with prevention and positive self-care. When diversity is devalued the potential for conveying these traits is compromised and poses a barrier to culturally competent care. Also, consumers are more likely to forego reporting for routine annual physical exams, psychoeducation, and other preventive procedures. Premature termination is also more likely to occur.

Relational theorists suggest that growth-fostering relationships empower by enlarging the capacities of those involved *to see the self and the other* more clearly and to act more progressively as a result of the connection created (Jenkins, 1995; Miller, 1976; Surrey, 1991, 1991a). Such relationships are facilitated by engagement, mutuality, empathy, and authenticity. Engagement is the ability to give attention and to express interest in another (Surrey, 1991b). Relative to pluralistic populations, it requires openness and flexibility in view of the collateral and affiliative values that are adhered to by these populations. Mutuality, an unconditional form of respect, is central to actualizing positive professional relationships given the disempowerment that many of these groups have suffered. Mutuality is open, reciprocal, and nonhierarchical. It is important for health and mental health providers in diverse communities to know that they have much to learn from consumers of care just as consumers of care can benefit from their expertise. Quality care delivery depends on collaborative effort. Empathy involves feeling with the consumer and is dependent on commonalties of human experience. Yet, Tyler, Brome, and Williams (1991) caution that ". . . commonality of experience cannot always be achieved" (p. 13). However, the practice of mutuality does much to compensate for any absence of empathy.

Authenticity is the ongoing challenge to feel "real," connected, vital, clear, and purposeful in relationship. It necessitates risk-taking and the willingness to challenge old images (Surrey, 1991) and practices. The personal qualities and practices that promote growth-fostering relationships, and the circumstances that contextualize such relationships vary from one reference group to another. These are dictated by cultural world views, values, social stratification, and the social history of a particular group in the United States.

Miller contends that "no culture provides an optimal relational context for living and developing because "[o]nce any group of people has been socially defined as dominant, and another as subordinate, there cannot be a full relational context" (p. 10). Therefore, the process of valuing diversity is a particular challenge for health and mental health providers who treat indigenous populations, for it challenges the essence of traditional practice as well as the dominant social order.

BARRIERS TO HELPSEEKING ON CAMPUS

In many ways communities are a cultural mosaic (Sue, 1992). Yet, many students of color who are in need of treatment never enter treatment at all, or enter treatment in crisis or with moderate to severe symptoms. Some terminate earlier in the treatment process than other students, have lower utilization rates, and lower positive outcome rates. Even though these patterns of utilization are not limited to students of color, the contexts to understanding them differ from those that underlie similar patterns for Caucasian, middle-class students. For students of color, these patterns of utilization are influenced in part by ethnocultural perceptions of helpseeking that differ from those of the dominant culture, the visibility of relatively few practitioners from same or similar backgrounds, and both the assumption and reality that some experienced practitioners have little or no empathy with, interests or competence in addressing psychosocial impacts of complex societal problems (e.g., racism, ethnocentrism, prejudice) or common racial and ethnic identity issues. Furthermore, college counselors and mental health practitioners are not always knowledgeable about enthnoculturally syntonic frameworks and considerations for care. Therefore, it is not surprising that some training sites fall short on preparing trainees to meet the needs of students of color effectively. For some college mental health facilities, readiness to serve diverse populations has become an even more complex issue due to the merger of services for students and managed care.

The College Mental Health Service as a Health Maintenance Organization: Troubling parallels between helpseeking in the community and on campus

Residents of inner city communities are often discouraged from seeking mental health care by a variety of barriers. For example, inadequate transportation, rotating staff, and dehumanizing features of public hospitals and clinics are among the structural barriers that have been identified in Chapter One. In addition, institutional/systemic barriers, which evolve from chronic societal problems include poverty, inadequate or the complete lack of health benefits, inability to negotiate the health care delivery system effectively, and inadequate health and psychoeducation. Social and ethnocultural barriers (e.g., prejudice, language differences, devaluation of cultural practices and lifestyles) result from lack of knowledge and familiarity with the ethnocultural backgrounds of people of color. A barrier imposed by the field of mental health in particular has been its tendency to overlook different cultural perceptions of mental health and mental illness rather than solely relying on perceptions based on medicocentric perspectives. These barriers are not as prevalent in college communities, but they do exist.

Some university health services provide care to students and employees. Some of these are also health maintenance organizations for employees and their families, and retired workers. For people of color in particular structural barriers often limit access to health and mental health care. For example, the wife of a service worker at a university reported irregularly for individual psychotherapy sessions citing transportation problems, and the therapist's lack of availability during evenings as reasons. Her health plan allowed a limited number of sessions on site and required a minimal copayment. The woman, an African Caribbean immigrant without a high school education, worked as a service worker on two stressful jobs over the course of several months of therapy. Getting time off to come for appointments became particularly difficult since she was also participating in family therapy sessions with her children once a week after school with another therapist at the same clinic. Much to her dissatisfaction, her husband refused to participate. Despite the scheduling conflict with her individual therapist, she refused to accept a referral to a therapist with more compatible hours despite relatively generous health benefits because she quickly became attached to the therapist, an African American woman, after she had agonized over beginning therapy. Also, she would not be able to afford the more costly 50% copayment that an outside referral would require. Needless to say, these difficulties did nothing to alleviate her depression, which was associated with childhood psychological and physical abuse, multiple losses associated with immigration, significant marital and family problems, and limited earning capacity. Eventually she dropped out of treatment despite persistent follow-up efforts.

This client represents an increasing population of those treated at college mental health facilitates that function also as managed care clinics. As more of these facilities also become components of health maintenance organizations, there will probably be an increase in clients, such as this Caribbean immigrant, who differ from traditional college students. The visibility of qualified therapists of color is particularly critical for some clients of color since it may communicate the possibilities to trust, to be understood, and to receive empathy. Based on this case example, it is also possible that despite significant problems in daily living and barriers to accessing care, a relationship with a therapist with at least some commonalties in social identity motivates some clients of color to remain in treatment longer than they would without this connection. Therefore, university health services–based health maintenance organizations must become more cognizant of the needs of nontraditional populations in order to attend to them effectively and to continue to attract a diverse consumer population.

CHALLENGES TO COLLEGE MENTAL HEALTH SERVICES

As the diversity of student populations increases to include more students of color, the field of college mental health faces some important challenges. First, standard theoretical and practice frameworks need to be modified in order to meet the needs of this steadily increasing population. Furthermore, in this era of managed care, time-limited and cost-effective care are essential. In addition, since colleges and universities have a profound influence on the communities that surround them, valuable opportunities exist for collaboration between university health and mental health resources and communities of color.

America's Heartland and Underserved Populations

Standard mental health care delivery systems have also neglected America's heartland, the Plains states and midwest, where all-

American lifestyles, beliefs, and values are strongly held, practiced, and influenced by a variety of ethnocultural nuances (regional, religious, bicultural) that do not necessarily support attention to psychological and social health. For example, one informal investigation into the availability of outpatient mental health resources in a diverse region of the Bible Belt revealed that there were few mental health providers prepared to treat people of color in that vicinity despite increasing evidence of psychological distress, somatic complaints, and social problems (violence and crime, substance abuse). Ethnic practices play a prominent role in shaping attitudes toward helpseeking. In view of the prominent role of churches in this particular region, perhaps community health psychologists could collaborate with church leaders and any local university health facilities in an effort to facilitate increased helpseeking in this region. To begin this process, psychoeducation workshops could be conducted at churches and/or open university forums which could eventually lead to more helpseeking. To expand on this example, churches could also become health networking sites and sources of grassroots participation in policymaking and governance. This is one of many examples of how community health psychologists could use the culture of a particular region as a guide or means for facilitating helpseeking for particular underserved populations.

PROGRESSIVE COLLABORATION

Collaborative efforts between university health providers and varied community resources have the potential to initiate progressive changes in communities of color. Such collaboration also has the potential of enhancing their status as institutions of knowledge and competence, while decreasing the elitist public image of some colleges and universities. Examples of such collaboration are evident in the Touchpoints Project and The Women in Prison Project.

The Touchpoints Project

The Touchpoints Project is a collaborative effort between the Brazelton Center for Infants and Parents (BCIP), a nonprofit arm of Children's Hospital in Boston, and psychologist consultants from the Stone Center at Wellesley College.

In the pilot phase of this project, psychologists trained pediatric nurse practitioners in developing positive relationships with young mothers from inner city areas. The rationale for this is that such relationships are critical to continuity of care for infants and toddlers. The training model integrates concepts from the relational theory of women's development (Jordan, Kaplan, Miller, et al., 1991) and social diversity theory (Chin, De La Cancela, & Jenkins, 1993) into a framework that facilitates the development of positive and mutually empowering relationships cross-culturally. A fundamental tenet of this model is that although the characteristics of positive and empowering relationships (i.e., engagement, empathy, authenticity, mutuality) are fairly consistent across cultures, the forms these take or the ways in which these are expressed, and appropriate ways of entering such relationships, are dictated by ethnocultural values and customs, and particular social histories of the reference groups, especially those circumstances that influenced their arrival. For example, for a Caucasian provider to initiate a new relationship with an African American mother by addressing her by her first name without first asking her permission to do so or how she would prefer to be addressed could be perceived by the mother as a sign of premature familiarity and disrespect. Therefore, it could interfere with the health provider's ability to engage and to establish an ongoing relationship with her. Because marital unions of African slave women were not taken seriously by those in power, and slaves were regarded as subhuman chattel, no formal titles (e.g., Miss, Mrs.) were used to address them. Some Caucasians have continued the practice over the centuries, perhaps without recognizing that it is, indeed, inappropriate, why this is so, and that it can have negative consequences for a positive working relationship.

The Touchpoints Project is intended to influence positive health care habits and wellness early in life via strengthening relationships between pediatric health practitioners and parents, some of whom are from inner city areas. Toward this end, parents are encouraged to bring infants and toddlers to clinics regularly for immunizations and periodic examinations. The Project also promotes positive relationships between new parents and their infants from the beginning of life by helping parents to recognize and to appreciate progress in the development of the infant. In this process, the focus on the baby by the health provider becomes a means of connecting with parents around the child's needs, listening to parents' concerns, and enlisting the collaboration of parents in the best interest of the child. Although the Touchpoints training model is still in its pilot phase, psychologists have been involved in developing and conducting this model.

The Women in Prison Project

The Women in Prison Project provides an example of how community health psychologists, state governing bodies on criminal justice, and minimum security women's prisons might collaborate effectively. This project was a fifteen-month endeavor funded by the Massachusetts Committee on Criminal Justice in collaboration with the Stone Center at Wellesley College to initiate an integrated relational and socially contextualized (Chin, De La Cancela, Jenkins, 1993) approach to the care and treatment of incarcerated women with an ultimate goal of reducing the depressive spiral that is commonly associated with substance abuse and criminal recidivism. Feminist scholars in the field of mental health have noted that this spiral includes social and emotional vulnerability, involvement in destructive relationships, and social isolation (Herman, 1991; Miller, 1976, 1986).

Psychologists were involved in all four phases of the Women in Prison Project. In phase one, the work of the Stone Center on women's relational development was introduced to administrators, staff, and post-release service providers. In the second phase, a series of focus groups and interviews with incarcerated women were conducted to assess their developmental histories, relational profiles, and their perceptions of their past and present needs. In phase three, interviews were conducted with staff for the purpose of developing a training framework based on concepts from relational theory and social diversity theory. The final phase involved creating, piloting, and evaluating that framework in a series of psychoeducation process groups with both staff and incarcerated women.

Relevance of Relational Theory and Social Diversity Theory for Women in Prison

The relational theory of women's development acknowledges that for women "the capacity to create meaningful relationships is the essence of development and psychological well-being" (Jordan, Kaplan, Miller, et al., 1991). Elsewhere this author contends that "openness to the diversity among women facilitates greater understanding of their strengths and the troublesome [conditions] that lead to [their involvement in] criminal activity (p. 17) (Jenkins, 1995). Such understanding is critical to psychological and social considerations for systematically reducing recidivism. Many incarcerated women are women of color. Many are also mothers, the carriers of culture. Without effective intervention, most are likely to pass on their self-defeating coping patterns to the next generation. Obviously, much is to be gained from modifying the relational patterns of incarcerated women. Prior to incarceration, many of these women had been deprived of the support systems and resources that might have prevented their becoming vulnerable to the societal problems that, for some, influenced low self-esteem and self-defeating coping strategies. Also, many of these women have suffered serious losses and violations (e.g., murdered loved ones, sexual trauma, abandonment, physical abuse) in primary relationships. A significant number of the crimes committed by the participants in the Women in Prison Project seemed to be symbolic of poor attempts to win or maintain the approval of a boyfriend or partner combined with the cumulative impact of involvement in unhealthy relationships over a period of several years.

Surrey's (1995) review of national data revealed that "a larger proportion of women than men involved with the criminal justice system are substance abusers. However, treatment programs for incarcerated women have been less available and most are not designed to meet women's particular needs and life circumstances" (p. 20). Many of the participants in the Women in Prison Project were recovering from substance abuse, trauma, and other psychological distress associated with chronic relational disconnections and violations suffered over the course of their lifetimes (Surrey, 1995). Furthermore, the onset of these conditions was often associated with self-defeating efforts to establish or maintain connection. For example, some women became involved in drug trafficking at the request of boyfriends or partners. Even though some women did not use drugs, they became involved in this illegal activity just to please their partners or to sustain the relationship. Others were introduced to substance abuse by these men. In several instances, not only did the substance abuse become established or maintain a connection to a significant other but in several cases it became a connection to life itself in the midst of pervasive isolation and abuse. In the latter cases, addiction obviously became a means of numbing the pain of everyday life.

THE IMPLICATIONS OF THE TOUCHPOINTS AND THE WOMEN IN PRISON PROJECTS FOR COMMUNITY HEALTH PSYCHOLOGISTS

The Touchpoints and the Women in Prison projects both illustrate the power of progressive collaboration between psychologists, health practitioners, and other human service professionals. Although both projects were quite different in purpose and populations served, each was oriented toward prevention and wellness. In addition, both projects recognized the centrality of growth-fostering relationships (i.e., personal and professional) to one's health status and overall well-being. Even though the Touchpoints Project was designed to include both parents and their infants, most of the parents and providers that actually participated were women. Of course, all of the group participants in the Women in Prison Project were women, while an appreciable number of the staff persons that participated in the training were men.

This author's consultation to both projects focused on helping them to deliver culturally competent intervention. Therefore, the design, execution, and evaluation of interventions were guided by sources of diversity. Efforts to respond to the specific health needs (physical, psychological, and social) of those served in a manner that felt relevant and helpful to them was primary. This required some specific knowledge of the providers and consumers served (family values, culture-specific health practices, economic realities) and appropriate ancillary resources in their communities. Of course, the role of consultant is only one of many to be assumed by community health psychologists. However, participation in the projects that have been described provides at least one window on the value of community health psychology as a specialty to the delivery of services that are compatible with the values, worldviews, and stated needs of clients. Moreover, the Stone Center's role as a university-based resource for these projects and the author's college mental health experience suggest that college mental health resources do, indeed, have meaningful roles to assume in promoting the physical, psychological, and social health in their surrounding communities at policy, governance, and service delivery levels.

COMMENTARY

Deborah Prothrow-Stith

In "Embracing People of Color: Implications for College Mental Health Services, " Yvonne Jenkins makes a strong and persuasive case for more culturally competent mental health services on college campuses. As traditionally white colleges become increasingly diverse, college mental health services have an ethical responsibility to review their methods of care and training in order to become inclusive of the needs of students of color and thus to remain a crucial and relevant resource for all college students. Dr. Jenkins comprehensively outlines the ways in which these services can and must embrace diversity.

If students of color are to feel comfortable turning to mental health services on campuses as a resource, then mental health professionals need to have empathy both for the psychosocial impacts of racial and ethnic identities, and for the ethnocultural perceptions of mental health care within different communities. Certain cultures, for example, do not uniformly categorize certain conditions as illnesses that require professional intervention. Mental health professionals also need to recognize the structural causes that may prevent a person of color from obtaining care. Without an awareness of ethnocultural issues, mental health practitioners are unable to effectively address the mental health needs of students of color.

Dr. Jenkins proposes that college mental health services engage in collaborative efforts with culturally competent community-based mental health resources that surround them in order to provide services that are accessible and sensitive to the needs of students of color. The recruitment of more minority mental health professionals on college campuses is critical to providing effective and appropriate care, as students of color may feel more comfortable with a practitioner who is of the same ethnocultural background.

Quality care delivery, Dr. Jenkins convincingly argues, depends on the provision of culturally competent care. Given the special developmental needs of college-age young adults, it is critical to an adequate college health system. But her call for a more culturally aware mental health system is also one that resonates beyond the parameters of college campuses and into our society at large.

SECTION III

TOWARD NEW MODELS

Reuben C. Warren

Health must embrace a more holistic view of well being, if new models of care for communities of color are expected. Even the classic definition of health used by the World Health Organization (WHO), the physical, social and psychological well-being of the individual, is too narrow. An internationally known black psychologist, Wade Nobles, describes health as a "relationship." Embracing the notion of a relationship, health can be described as "a dynamic relationship focused on the physical, social, psychological, and spiritual well-being of the individual and/or group and their interaction with the physical and social environment." This definition does not include disease in its scope.

Expanding on the definition from WHO, three essential elements evolve: The group, spirituality, and the social and physical environments. These three elements are particularly important in communities of color for several reasons. First, it is unlikely that any system of care will be effective if the individual is viewed in isolation from their group. The group dynamic, be it immediate or extended family, community or race/ethnic identification, is foundational in communities of color. Second, the role of spirituality in health and health care delivery is increasingly recognized by the public health community. Spirituality focuses on meaning and value, which have been major challenges for communities of color in their historic evolution in U.S. culture. And third, the role of social and physical environment has an ever-growing role in health and health care, particularly for communities of color.

The role of psychology, particularly ethnocultural psychology, will allow primary care and other health strategies to embrace this expanded definition in ways which will enhance the delivery of care. Although the role of human behavior in sustaining health has not been fully recognized, it is clear that current threats to health are driven by social, behavioral, economic, cultural, and political factors. The biological outcomes, such as illness, sickness, disability, and premature death are merely failures of the social system.

New models must be amenable to the rigor of public health science, while at the same time, they must not only use the traditional outcome measures of success, such as the reduction in morbidity and mortality. Health is confounded by far too many factors outside of the health delivery system to measure success by these traditional criteria. Measures of effort, performance, adequacy of performance, efficacy and process are also needed. Only if the group's well-being is enhanced will the long-term health of individuals in communities of color be sustained. The importance of the group does not ignore the realities of the health status of the individual or the need for curative care. However, the group dynamic requires that other salient issues be considered related to community health in planning, implementing and evaluating care models.

Lifestyle changes are being stressed by public health experts as an area for health improvement. However, new models for health and health care must also address the circumstance of the individual or group. "Life circumstance" is a convenient way to describe all the factors that have historically and continuously influenced the social and physical environment in which one finds herself. For example, billboards advertising tobacco and alcohol are disproportionately located in communities of color and the promotion of violence by the popular media, adversely influence smoking and alcohol use as antisocial behavior. The negative depiction of people of color, particularly African American youth, surely influence decision making for many young people. While these matters may not fit the classic definition of risk factors, one must acknowledge their probable influence on human behavior.

The theory and practice of behavioral sciences are essential to success in primary care even though the principles of the behavioral sciences have not always been acknowledged by primary care providers. Yet, the behavioral constraints such as beliefs, belief systems, values, perception, and cultural competence form the basis for effective communication in health care delivery.

Finally, the foundational model for community health psychology must embrace health promotion as an entity distinct from disease prevention. Disease prevention assumes that one will get sick. The efforts are to identify risk factors and/or disease as early as possible and design interventions for prevention. Alternatively, one can view health as a normal phenomenon and disease, disability, and premature death as abnormal. A proactive health promotion strategy may then evolve. Health is normal! People don't have to get sick! The question which will then drive the strategy is "What have we done to deviate from the normal and how do we design systems to return to health?"

With the current poor health status in many communities of color, it is difficult to envision health as normal. However, unless this vision is embraced, the old models of care will be reconfigured with new buzz words. The current health disparities based on race and/or ethnicity, regardless of income or education, will continue. We must design new models, test those models, affirm their efficacy and "Expect Miracles."

9

Diversity in Community Health Psychology: Toward New Models

Victor De La Cancela, Jean Lau Chin, and Yvonne M. Jenkins

WHY COMMUNITY HEALTH PSYCHOLOGY?

Currently organized psychology is struggling to have its health service provider roles more clearly acknowledged by health service consumers, payors of health services, employers, and by psychologists themselves (Suinn, 1996). For all stakeholders, accomplishing such recognition requires a shift in the traditional clinical psychology paradigm to include a health psychology focus, community psychology orientation, organizational change perspective, and cultural competency. We believe that combining the various approaches of community and clinical psychology with the recent advances of public health practice in diverse communities is necessary to achieve health promotion, disease prevention, service delivery, and professional training that addresses the complex sociopolitical issues of power and change in communities of color. We embark from our previous collaboration on integrating socioeconomic, historical, ethnoracial, and gender contexts into more traditional notions of psychotherapy and mental health to a contemporary expansion of psychology's contribution to community health policy concerns in practice, research, and service delivery systems design. Relying upon our extensive clinical and administrative experience in community mental health and community health as well as teaching and independent practice, we ask systemic, "interruptive" questions that psychologists and other behavioral health professionals can consider to fashion interdisciplinary and systemic approaches to specific social health problems extant among diverse communities.

Most health psychology publications emphasize a narrow practice of psychology within health care settings, and relegate psychology to a supportive role. Health psychology has generally meant the application of psychology in medical settings to dying patients, psychosomatic illnesses, or serious medical illnesses. It has not been generally applied to examine systems of care. Given rapid changes in our health care delivery systems, the need for relevant models which are inclusive of all segments of the population is both cost effective and ethically responsible. We propose an expanded role for psychologists within health care settings which will become increasingly important in a population-based managed health environment. The role of community health psychologists will enable psychologists as administrators and health service providers to contribute to health policy, public health, and health care services delivery by emphasizing that the diverse health-related needs of communities of color must be met more effectively (Smith & Anderson, 1990). In addition, effective systems of health care must be shaped by an integrative perspective of the communities where people of color live. With movement toward change through embracing diversity, community health psychologists further expand the definition of psychology to be inclusive of health, and the interaction of health needs, and systems of health care.

A key principle of community health psychology is to expand and link the contextual and sociopolitical aspects and realities of communities to their health experiences, thereby setting the stage for a progressive health psychology that explores and challenges the status quo as part of the service delivery process; for professional advocacy that challenges psychologists to reexamine their role and function as change agents; and for a multidisciplinary, multicultural perspective that requires collaboration among health professionals, healers, and consumers of varied sociopolitical and psychocultural world views. As in our earlier book, *Diversity in psychotherapy: The politics of race, ethnicity, and gender* (Chin, De La Cancela, & Jenkins, 1993), we attempt to make conscious the broad historical context and political aspects of the health status of our communities, and choose to make our values and biases apparent.

Our individual perspectives not only come from the personal, ethnic, and professional experiences which influenced the content of each chapter, these individual approaches also reflect both the diversity and shared vision of a community health model. Specifically, they reflect Dr. De La Cancela's study of the importance of sociopolitical factors and socioeconomic context in health care theory, practice, outcomes, and systems, as well as his training, expertise, and commitment to cognitive, psychoeducational, and community health education approaches that transfer knowledge toward self-care and well-being. Drs. De La Cancela and Chin evolved into community health psychology by developing interest and experiences in school psychology, mental retardation and learning disabilities, primary care, substance abuse prevention and treatment, community competence and empowerment, and policymaking and administration. Dr. Chin trained in a research oriented program, worked in a child guidance clinic for 15 years with a psychodynamic orientation, yet used her school psychology training to bring a cognitive-behavioral perspective to clinical practice. Her ethnic identification and perspective ultimately integrated with her professional perspective to blend systemic, cultural, psychodynamic, and cognitive contributions into a personalized clinical practice and administration approach. Dr. Jenkins's metamorphosis into community health psychology stems from psychoeducation and counseling perspectives, long years of independent practice, vocational rehabilitation and employee assistance program consultation, and service provider expertise. Her early work focused on identifying and advocating for homebound mentally retarded African American children who were neglected by service delivery systems. Thereafter, her vocational rehabilitation expertise targeted special needs inner city students and adults with severe mental illness. Considerable experience in college mental health, research on community crisis intervention, and her social identity have blended into a theory and practice which integrates systemic, cultural, psychodynamic, cognitive-behavioral, and relational components. We have become community health psychologists by transforming our roles as psychologists, administrators, and policymakers and advocating for systemic and infrastructure changes through a community health psychology praxis which empowers communities, promotes access, and improves the health of the community. We believe such transformation is necessary for the empowerment of diverse communities in their comprehensive struggles to prevent chronic illnesses, infectious disease, and social pathologies.

In the creation of a culturally competent health care system, the error of exclusion is fatal, i.e., excluding a significant but minority segment of the population. We recognize the limitations of this book in not including a Native American perspective. As persons of color from East Coast cities, our perspectives are limited not only by our ethnicities and racial identifications, but also by geography and urban perspectives. Our omissions do not reflect a failure to value the diversity within the U.S. population, or a political faux pas of excluding one of four significant national minority populations within the United States. Rather, we felt the biases and values inherent in our cultural, professional, personal, and ethnic experiences reflect the contextual and sociopolitical realities of our communities, which is not inclusive of all perspectives. We chose not to write about that which we did not experience, especially where significant differences might violate the uniqueness within American Indian communities. Ours was not an attempt to exclude but to reflect our limited perspectives and to respect the right of other communities to speak with their own voices. In so doing, we hope to demonstrate, as an underlying premise, the need for flexibility and outer directedness in any system or perspective. This premise, essential to a community health psychology model, enables a system to modify itself to meet the unique needs of diverse groups.

REDEFINING COMMUNITY-ORIENTED PRIMARY CARE

In this transformation, several themes emerge to challenge existing concepts, and to promote new models. Historically, clinical-community psychologists have much insight and expertise to offer in the area of increasing access and delivery of community oriented health care services to diverse populations, based upon the myriad issues they have confronted in providing psychological care to poor and underserved communities in community health centers and community mental health centers. Such community health centers (CHC) have shouldered the brunt of services to a disproportionate number of Medicaid clients and diverse racial and ethnic populations. Access to care for communities of color is still lacking, however, due to language and cultural incompatibility between CHC providers and some ethnoracial subgroups as well as barriers such as citizenship requirements and racism. Toward promoting change in the context of a changing health care environment, we outline some of the remedies we believe need to be made in order to improve the delivery of primary care. Mention is also made of innovative community health programs that can be developed to address some of the psychological and cultural influences reviewed earlier. Changes must be made at different levels and on different fronts within the areas of graduate education in psychology and health, legislative and funding initiatives, health policy directives, recruitment, retention and training of health care professionals and establishing partnerships. Ultimately, community empowerment must be achieved.

As health systems reforms emphasize cost containment and managed care, we face new challenges in developing community oriented primary care. Most large health systems confront psychosocial and cultural issues daily in addition to coping with drastic budget reductions, elimination of positions, and the challenges of managed care. These reductions increase waiting time for appointments, waiting time to fill prescriptions, pressure on providers to see more patients while clinic hours are reduced, and pressure on emergency rooms. They also foster the development of higher copayments for clients. Staff reductions often include facility support staff (i.e., housekeeping, dietary, security, and maintenance) and administrative positions; they are usually part of overall downsizing and other cost-cutting mechanisms to reduce the ever-increasing cost of providing health care. As a result, many health systems are confronting an unprecedented challenge: How do we build a community-oriented primary care system in the face of diminishing resources?

Community-oriented primary care (COPC) combines traditional primary care with public health services and education such as immunizations and infectious disease control. To expand professional psychology's contribution to this process as a health service requires a resurgence of interest in community psychology and a more applied focus to health psychology. The interface between psychology and health is significant given that mind and body, psychological health and physical health are interconnected. This connection is dramatically seen in instances of somatization, where personal and social distress is manifested in bodily complaints and health care-seeking behavior. Studies estimate that 40 to 60% of primary care visits have psychological origins. Traditional biomedical models lead to the underdiagnosis of these psychosocial problems, neglect of their impact on health and mental health status, and the utilization of expensive and unnecessary laboratory analysis and physician services rather than psychological treatment. Traditional clinical psychology and clinical health psychology approaches can remedy some of the shortcomings of biomedical models by attending to cognitive, behavioral, and lifestyle factors; yet, they too often adhere to disease treatment and curative models that at best are secondary prevention and tertiary intervention. Community psychology offers an environmental perspective, primary prevention interventions in schools, occupational and other institutional settings, and focus on action research and issues of power and change. It poses systemic, "interruptive " questions, though it has not been traditionally defined as a health service delivery model.

Combining these perspectives into a comprehensive community health psychology approach in primary care service delivery would lead to both more person centered and systemic models which lessen the fragmentation of the patient and care provided to her. Compliance and recovery issues, placebo effects, health beliefs and behavior, and communication styles are all highly influenced by social, cultural, and psychological factors that include individual health status, ethnoracial group membership, community stressors, socioeconomic resources, familial supports, and access to health care. Table 9.1 provides some examples of barriers to comprehensive and more culturally inclusive health service delivery that are generated by agencies or individual clinicians.

The identified obstacles below reflect a lack of diversity and lack of cultural competence in that they characterize professionals and organizations who treat everyone in the same manner. This usually translates to serving only the majority or mainstream groups best. The views of health and diagnosis that emerge from these generally traditional approaches to health care depend upon: denial of ethnic specific differences; nonegalitarian labelling; intrapsychic orientations; allegedly apolitical and sociohistorically noncontextualized interpretation; lack of ethnocultural self-awareness; conservatism and fears of admitting ignorance for fear of rejection from mainstream health care. In short, these approaches provide narrow views of health, reflect chauvinistic and ethnocen-

TABLE 9.1

CLINICAL/INSTITUTIONAL BARRIERS TO SERVICE DELIVERY

Language differences	Class bound values
Ethnocentrism	Monocultural assumptions
Racism	Heterosexism
Prejudice	Dominant culture preferences
Countertransference	Color blindness
Biomedical models	Office bound
Lack of evening hours	Home visits not offered
Bureaucracy	Scientific reductionism
Professionalism	Nondirective approaches
Deficit-focused	Individualistic bias
Victim-blaming	Xenophobia
Generalizations	Stereotypes
Rigid family definitions	Managed Care

tric expectations, overvalue the status quo, and follow the path of least social resistance.

Community health psychology attempts to be more comprehensive and inclusive by addressing health needs through empowerment, improving individual health status through combined individual-community interventions, and overcoming service barriers with culturally competent access. It involves health promotion, health education and prevention, psychoeducation, psychological counseling and community consultation, program design, implementation and evaluation, and advocacy, research, and administration. It is a conscious departure from the micro, laboratory, and research settings of traditional health psychology to the public services field of promotion, prevention, and advocacy and policymaking in response to systemic gaps and barriers in the mainstream health care delivery system. Primary to various community health psychology interventions is a commitment to influence public health policy, improve systems of care, and provide community-based service delivery for all participants in care.

DEVELOPING NEW PARTNERSHIPS

Most psychologists working in community health centers and community mental health centers have extensive backgrounds of working in teams that include the disciplines of nursing, social work, public health, psychiatry, and primary care. Thus, they have a biopsychosocial appreciation of the patient's world. If nothing more, psychologists have been successful in utilizing an ecostructural-systems approach that recognizes the importance of partnership.

They have "networked" with private nonprofit human service organizations, with academia and other research organizations, and they have done this with the recognition of their interdependence. Yet, psychologists must also establish major collaborative relationships with community-based organizations, activists, advocates, and gatekeepers, unions, and local and state governmental officials to leverage outside funding for programs beneficial to disenfranchised populations. Nutritional counseling, crime reduction, youth and family services, day care and transportation programs must be included as providers of wraparound and support services within community health psychology approaches, managed care networks, and other health care delivery models. In advocating for such services, community health psychologists will be meeting a societal responsibility to promote the availability of resources that allow health choices to be made freely, intelligently, and within the consumer's preferred residential or occupational networks.

DEFINING CULTURALLY COMPETENT SYSTEMS

We view cultural competence as a developmental goal and process toward which psychologists, other behavioral scientists, agencies, institutions, and systems can strive. In community health psychology, cultural competence includes valuing diversity, continuous self-examination, intercultural consciousness, institutionalized cultural knowledge and resources, various adaptations of service models to better meet patient needs, and input from communities of color and diverse constituencies. Workers in culturally competent systems have both the will and capacity to assist diverse communities; they acknowledge that race, gender, culture, and ethnicity make a difference and that all people are not, nor should they be, the same. These systems attend to cultural strengths, seek to deliver quality services, attempt to improve upon systemic weaknesses, add to their knowledge base and advocate for equitable practices, policies, and application of resources. What follow are some of the crosscutting issues which culturally competent systems of care might concern themselves with.

Graduate Health Education

One of community health psychology's major goals is to diversify clinical training from specialized mental health services to community oriented primary psychological health care. Currently, there is a shortage of physicians, psychologists, and other health care providers committed to practicing community responsive primary health care, the result of a health profession's education system which continues to focus on specialization, while increasingly, the U.S. population has limited access to primary care (Smith & Anderson, 1990). To change this approach, medical schools, doctoral psychology programs, and public health programs should be exploring ways to move the graduate health classroom into the community (Smith & Anderson, 1990). While such efforts are gradual, over time they can alter the reputation of graduate health schools as social organizations that are resistant to change (Bloom, 1989). This would enable them to make more meaningful contributions to the overall well being of the community than in the past.

Crosscutting education combining the various approaches of community and clinical psychology with new advances in public health and primary care can be fashioned in predoctoral practicum and internship programs and at the postdoctoral fellowship, residency, and continuing education levels. More interdisciplinary collaboration with social work, medical sociology, health education, substance abuse counseling, and clinical anthropology would move psychology toward greater adherence to espoused holistic and biopsychosocial models (Abramson & Kark, 1983).

More specifically, the doctoral psychology curriculum must be expanded to include the subject areas of public health: health policy, disease prevention, biostatistics, surveillance, epidemiology, health ethics, community health education, and community organization.

Recruitment and Retention

COPC faces significant challenges in overcoming the "convenience factor" to which some health professionals have become accustomed; that is to say, the convenience of working in hospitals or in offices in close proximity to hospitals (Smith, Brooks, & Anderson, 1991). However, the convenience of 9 to 5 work/office hours, Monday through Fridays, is seldom the best for patients. Communities of color need primary care clinicians who are willing to work in the community and are committed to staying there and developing long-lasting relationships with their patients. Clearly, rhetoric far outdistances practice in this regard.

While psychology's efforts are to be commended, we need to do more to recruit and retain culturally competent, skilled health care providers. Specifically, organized psychology needs to fund programs that encourage cultural sensitivity, understanding, and competence and provide ongoing training and proficiency and specialty certification to assist providers to appropriately staff intake and assessment, counseling, vocational and educational training, and health psychology centers. Health education, peer support group co-facilitation, and forensic, legal, immigration, and housing mediation and advocacy are some of the necessary skills needed by providers to fully assume the role of health care professionals who are providing culturally competent care that promotes health, prevents disease, and improves treatment outcomes and overall health and mental health status. This new provider will serve the multiple health and human service needs of individuals whose health and welfare are especially at risk. A major need among communities of color is the tremendous shortage of psychiatrists and primary care doctors who are appropriately trained and can prescribe, monitor, and regulate psychotropic medication and provide culturally competent psychotherapy in rural and inner city areas or state correctional and mental retardation/developmental disabilities facilities. Thus, proficiency and specialty training for psychologists in prescribing and administering psychotropic medication is also needed to ensure that cost-effective and quality psychopharmacological and psychotherapeutic services are provided to patients of color.

Legislative and Funding Initiatives

Funding at the federal, state, and local levels is also changing to reflect a policy toward developing primary care and preventive services rather than tertiary care. Future primary care services and related expenditures should therefore involve psychological service centers shifting their priorities to internally fund primary care programs as well as applying for and receiving funding for specific primary care initiatives.

For example:

- Behavioral health centers can develop comprehensive adolescent services, address physical-mental health conditions (such as anger and trauma management) and drug abuse services. Services for adult trauma victims are also needed.
- Psychological services centers can implement case and disease management for asthmatic children, cardiac patients, migraine sufferers, diabetics, and hypertensives in primary care services who can also be followed on the inpatient side.
- Mental health centers can add evening hours or weekend morning hours, and 24-hour coverage in primary psychological care to meet the criteria for managed care programs.

Community based psychologists can secure and obtain new funding for:

- providing integrated comprehensive health care services for adolescent health in junior high and middle schools. Psychologists can stress disease prevention/health promotion and serve as a conduit for referral to specialty services provided elsewhere;
- implementing primary care services for substance using women, their children, and significant others, expanding clinic hours to evenings and weekends, and adding selected specialty-subspecialty services in order to decompress hospital emergency rooms;
- supportive services for new parents such as parenting classes, stress management, and counseling.

Recognizing that psychological care must often be delivered in the context of primary care and specialized services, we can develop programs that attempt to meet our patients' health care needs. This might involve effective collaboration with other health professionals and inclusion of psychologists as family-oriented health care professionals in legislation addressing primary care. Besides increasing services for HIV/AIDS related psychological care at off-site facilities, we can target adolescents and adults who reside in disenfranchised communities in an effort to reduce the risk of HIV infection. The linkage between primary care, psychological care, and substance abuse is critical to providing appropriate treatment. Some programs use acupuncture as an adjunct to more conventional medical and psychiatric services. Other special populations such as women, children of substance abusers, probationers, persons with HIV/AIDS, and teenage or new parents will also require developmentally and culturally competent and supportive psychological services.

As the principal sources of health care for the working poor, community health systems are the most appropriate place to develop a psychological model of care for this population that will integrate occupational health and primary care services. Additionally, there are many opportunities for psychologist-primary care practitioner collaboration in migrant, rural, and homeless health centers to develop and document community health models of service delivery that can be replicated in other communities.

Resources will also be needed to successfully implement Medicaid and Medicare Managed Care. Managed care presents community health psychologists with an opportunity to provide primary care for poor and elderly patients, only if patients have the educational resources to appropriately utilize all the essential components of a managed care system. Psychologists can work with health systems to develop plans for managed care and as part of this effort, increase the number of patients who appropriately utilize their specific provider in the primary care clinic by expanding their knowledge of the health system. Educational empowerment of staff by psychologists allows outpatient departments to provide greater continuity of relevant patient care and is critical for enhanced patient participation in Medicaid and Medicare Managed Care programs.

COMMUNITY EMPOWERMENT

Community-oriented primary care requires the employment of multidisciplinary health care professionals of color and others with varied language proficiencies. Many community health centers are staffed largely by and for low income communities and communities of color. Urban health facilities are also major economic forces in the communities they serve, many of which are poor. Thus, institutional leadership must not only reflect its communities, but use its economic power as well, to build these communities and offer economic opportunity to their residents.

Psychologist-administrators can play a major role in leading such institutions by sharing their expertise and vast knowledge with others. In psychology, we have several health related specialties including rehabilitation psychology, health psychology, medical psychology, clinical psychology, counseling psychology, clinical neuropsychology, pediatric psychology, school psychology, physiological psychology, and psychopharmacology, as well as consulting and organizational/industrial psychologists in health care management who can be useful in this regard. Psychology also has a long tradition of attending to social and policy issues, organizational change and law, and business and consumer behavior which can be realigned in the service of empowering consumers and communities toward total health. A sampling of the necessary leadership includes: opposition to exclusionary legislation aimed at legal immigrants; increasing resources for ethnic- and race-specific health service delivery; promotion of bilingual/bicultural health care programs and research; identifying gaps in disease prevention and health promotion data, for communities of color, people with low incomes, people with disabilities, and people of diverse sexual orientations; and establishing education and public information programs to reduce health risks.

This call for community health empowerment and psychology's role in it are what makes this book and our elaboration of themes and issues different from what has come before. Ultimately, we are calling for the integration of psychology's clinical/service, applied research, and basic research specialties in the interest of the public's health. Terms such as community-oriented primary care are not new; nor are diversity and empowerment. Moreover, managed care and health reform are debated and developed within the mainstream. Our community health psychology approach is a way of taking existing concepts, and building and expanding them for the next century. Moreover, this approach takes what is happening in the mainstream, and ensures that whatever form health reform and managed care take, it will be relevant and inclusive of communities of color and will value the diversity of our population. Otherwise we could repeat the mistakes that have kept groups and communities disenfranchised and underserved. This is not only a moral, ethical issue; it is also one of cost, be it measured in the number of lives needlessly lost or dollars expended in treating preventable conditions after they have become acute or chronic.

The National Empowerment Center (Bureau, 1993) has identified some paths to mental health consumer/psychiatric survivor empowerment that community health empowerment can follow as well: full access to information about the side effects of medications, the reality of recovery from illness and disease, what works and what strategies have really improved the quality of life; full informed consent about specific drugs and treatments, and genuine alternatives and practical coping skills that have been utilized effectively in place of standard biomedical methods; information on support groups and self-help networks for health consumers to share their valuable experience and learning with others; the existence of government benefits and civil rights protection such as the Americans with Disabilities Act and advance directives, proxy agreements, or living wills in multiple languages; and the consumer's right to contact administrators, government officials, and policymakers directly if he experiences abuse, neglect, or incompetence while under the care of the health systems for which these officials are accountable.

Community health empowerment means that community residents have learned to find their own voices and the strength of their collective experiences, and are able to understand the power of anger, especially when it is channeled in ways that create long-term social change by challenging patterns of systematic discrimination in medical care and health education for the betterment of all in society (Bureau, 1993). Once empowerment is experienced by a community or individual, they commit themselves to it, for it means having a good understanding of the barriers and getting access to the tools and strategies needed to create a better quality of life.

CONCLUSION

In closing, we emphasize that one cannot lose sight of the enormity of the task before us. Just as describing the excesses of a hospital oriented and medicocentric health care system in a few pages is a challenge, so is it a challenge to refrain from seeking a quick solution. We must recognize that psychology for several years has been codependent and enabling of an acute care and specialty oriented system that has contributed to the present shortages in primary care. We must engage in strategic planning, diagnosis and treatment, management, and program evaluation by setting realistic objectives, ensuring fiscal accountability, and acknowledging the wisdom provided by the front liners—those in the community—rather than management influenced by guild interests or by professional careers.

For those of you willing to engage in that long hard struggle, community health psychology welcomes your efforts. For those of you not yet convinced, we ask that you channel your skepticism into collaborative challenges that improve our knowledge of innovative, creative, and long-standing interventions.

COMMENTARY
Toward a Pedagogy of
Community Health Psychology

Bertha Garrett Holliday

In the previous chapter, the book's authors articulated a visionary perspective of the need for and concerns of community health psychology. They also described the pathways of their personal "evolution" into community health psychologists, which involved continuing efforts to effect some synthesis of their cultural sensibilities and values, their professional skills, and the needs and demands of the organizations and communities where they worked. Such evolution is a reinventive process that is incremental, dialectical, inclusionary, organic—and may include unexpected detours in one's professional career path. Nevertheless, it is a process that is amenable to at least partial replication through professional training and socialization processes that involve: (a) a pedagogy that is grounded in individual and institutional commitments to lifelong learning in multiple settings, and (b) models of practice, research, and program evaluation that serve to develop and guide both that new knowledge of health in diverse populations and those innovative health services and systems that are required by a community health psychology.

In January 1977, the American Psychological Association's Commission on Ethnic Minority Recruitment, Retention, and Training in Psychology identified the following five models of education and training in multicultural issues, which I believe are also supportive of community health psychology: (a) models for ensuring that all future psychologists develop some minimal competence in multicultural issues; (b) models that seek to prepare professionals to provide services to linguistically diverse populations; (c) models that value ethnic minority professionals and communities; (d) models that promote specialized competence in multicultural issues; and (e) models that emphasize applied and community-based research in ethnic minority communities.

Furthermore, I would like to suggest that doctoral programs aspiring to train community health psychologists would be characterized by:

1) concentrated coursework in a major clinical or biomedical area within the discipline of psychology;

2) multidisciplinary coursework outside the discipline of psychology;

3) *continuous practicum experiences in a range of community settings serving diverse populations;*

4) *provision of structured opportunities where "success" is dependent on collaborative (preferably multidisciplinary) group effort;*

5) *involvement in training programs and community agencies and institutions that actively seek to continuously evolve and modify their training and service approaches in response to the needs of a pluralistic society, related new knowledge, and changing marketplaces; and*

6) *training in research and evaluation approaches that are responsive to: (a) the transformations of health care marketplaces, services systems, and diverse groups; (b) differences in health status, symptomatology, and treatment outcomes among and within diverse groups; and (c) health economics modeling techniques that facilitate comparisons among communities and cultural groups.*

Training of this type will seek to socialize professionals for practice, professional development, and lifelong learning that are characterized by a willingness to: (a) adopt culturally diverse perspectives and multidisciplinary technologies; (b) value multiple ways of "knowing" and embrace multiple simultaneous realities; (c) assess problems and strengths at multiple levels of etiology and impact including intrapsychic/biological, behavioral/medical, family, community, cultural group, institutional; and (d) adapt and reinvent one's professional role and activities through continual development of new competencies in response to new challenges.

Such a pedagogical model is necessary if community health psychology is to attain and maintain the promise so enthusiastically described by the book's authors.

AFTERWORD

Arthur Kleinman

This book is a practical guide for the clinician, the health program administrator, and the community mental health planner. It provides conceptual frameworks, models, and practical guidelines for how to engage diversity in community mental health settings. It is written by experienced mental health professionals who have made a mark in the mental health field serving underserved ethnic populations.

Heretofore cultural competence, diversity training, and community programs for ethnic groups were all seen as a specialty area of cultural psychiatry or psychology. But things are changing, demographically and in the mental health field. We are increasingly aware of the growth of racial and ethnic diversity in North American society. That more than half the United States population will be members of such ethnic groups a half century from now means that we are at ground zero. From here on year by year, the issues reviewed in this text will become increasingly mainstreamed. They will be part of the core competencies mental health professionals of all types will be expected to master; and they will hold high salience.

I have worked in this field for three decades. It is hard for me to understand the full significance of the reality I am describing, because I have long experienced the marginalization of cultural perspectives and sources of knowledge. But epochs change, and ours is going through an enormous transformation with respect to issues of diversity. That change means that the materials covered in this book will be widely read. To help make them more accessible I wish to frame them with several large conceptual concerns.

First, if cultural approaches are to be practicable, effective, and not misused, we need to specify when culture is salient and when it is not in mental health settings. Obviously, for patients and clients from ethnic minority and refugee groups, culture is usually important in clinical care. But it is also essential to recognize that culture is usually regarded as important with economically disadvantaged, underserved populations. In those groups and communities, economic factors are at least as significant as cultural ones. Indeed, too often in such settings attention to a client's cultural issues may mask poverty, unemployment, and other economic factors that need to be addressed. Thus, concern for cultural competence must also include concern for economic influences on health, illness, and care.

Second, culture as a practical concept must be broadened to include examination of how the professional culture of mental health providers and the particular cultural ethos of the institutions within which they practice affect caregiving. In my own clinical experience, the culture of the provider is as significant a source of obstacles to effective care as the culture of the family and patient.

Third, in the general society one of the most profound cultural effects is racism. It influences mental health problems, their course and outcome, and their treatment. Mental health providers cannot change racism in society, but they can establish procedures in the bureaucratic settings in which they work to make sure that racism and its pernicious effects are regularly assessed and dealt with.

Fourth, the American Psychiatric Association's DSM-IV includes a useful methodology for routinely engaging culture. Regrettably, it is currently buried in this hefty tome's ninth appendix. This clinically applied methodology should be included in courses on cultural competence. It includes four steps in the evaluation process for any mental health problem:

1) Attend to clear identification of the patient's ethnic, subethnic, and cultural background; and determine in what ways that background is immediately relevant for the problem at hand.
2) Evaluate cultural meanings and practices such as idioms of distress or culturally salient syndromes that influence the diagnostic and treatment process via solicitation of the patient's and family's explanatory models of illness and narratives of the illness experience. (For details see Kleinman, 1988, 1996; Mezzich et al, 1996.)
3) Evaluate influence of cultural processes on experiences of support and stress (axes four and five of the DSM's axial system of diagnoses).
4) Relate these and other factors (e.g., ethnopsychopharmacological effects) in treatment process.

This methodology fits rather well, it seems to me, within the broad array of approaches to cultural competence outlined in this volume.

References

Abramson, J.H., & Kark, S.L. (1983). Community oriented primary care: Meaning and scope. In E. Connor & F. Mullan (Eds.). *Community oriented primary care: New directions for health services delivery. Conference proceedings.* Washington, DC: Institute of Medicine.

Action for Primary Care Legislation. (1993). *Righting the health care pyramid: The need for a New York State primary conversion plan.* New York: Action for Primary Care Legislation.

Aday, L.A. (1993). *At Risk in America.* San Francisco: Jossey-Bass Inc.

Alder, H.M., & Hammett, V.B.O. (1973). The doctor-patient relationship revisited: An analysis of the placebo effect. *Annals of Internal Medicine, 78,* 595–598.

American Psychological Association. (1997). *American Psychologist, 52,* (2).

Appel, F., & Dunn, C. (1993). Process improvement: New health care landscape places premium on quality tools. *Total Quality Newsletter, 4* (11), 5.

Asian American Health Forum. (1990). *Fact sheets: A/PI: Dispelling the myth of a healthy minority.* San Francisco: APIAHF.

Association of Asian Pacific Community Health Organizations. (1993). *Lifting barriers to Asian and Pacific health care: Issues and recommendations.* Oakland, CA: Association of Asian Pacific Community Health Organizations, Asian American Health Forum, National Asian Pacific American Families Against Substance Abuse, and GAPA Community HIV Project.

Baer, H.A. (1986). Towards a critical medical anthropology. *Social Science and Medicine, 23,* 95–98.

Barbarin, O. A., Good, P. R., Pharr, O. M., & Siskind, J. A. (1981). *Institutional racism and community competence.* Washington, DC: Superintendent of Documents, U.S. Government Printing Office.

Barker, J. C. (1992). Cross-cultural medicine: A decade later. Cultural diversity—Changing the context of medical practice. *The Western Journal of Medicine, 157* (3), 248–254.

Bass, B.A., Wyatt, G.E., & Powell, G.J. (1982). *The Afro-American: Assessment, treatment and research issues.* New York: Grune & Stratton.

Becker, D., Lira, E., & Castillo, M. I. (1990). Therapy with victims of political repression in Chile: The challenge of social reparation. *Journal of Social Issues, 46* (3), 133–149.

Bellevue Hospital Center. (1993, May 27). *The Leadership Bulletin.* New York: Bellevue Hospital Center Public Affairs Department.

Blendon, R. J., Marttila, J., Benson, J. M., Shelter, M. C., Connoly, F. J., & Kiley, T. (1994). Health care reform. *Health Affairs, 13* (1), 274–284.

Bloom, S.W. (1989). The medical school as a social organization: The sources of resistance to change. *Medical Education, 23* (3), 228–241.

Boston At Risk 2000. (1994). *Six principles for a new health care system: A blueprint for action.* Boston: Families USA.

Boston Persistent Poverty Project. (1989). *In the midst of plenty.* Boston: Author.

Bowser, B., Arietta, G., & Jones, T. (1993). *Confronting diversity on campus.* Newbury Park, CA: Sage.

Boyle, P. J., & Callahan, D. (1993). Minds and hearts: Priorities in mental health services. *Hastings Center Report, 23* (5), S3–23.

Brazelton, T. B. (1992). *Touchpoints.* Reading, MA: Addison-Wesley.

Breckon, D.J., Harvey, J.R., & Lancaster, R.B. (1989). *Community health education: Settings, roles, and skills.* Gaithersburg, MD: Aspen.

Brennfleck Pascuzzi, E. (1993). Claims and benefits administration. In P.R. Kongstvedt (Ed.). *The managed health care handbook.* Gaithersburg, MD: Aspen.

Brockway, J. (1980). Pain and its management: A behavioral-medicine perspective. In N. Jospe, J. Nieberding & B.D. Cohen (Eds.). *Psychological factors in health care* (pp. 169–183). Lexington, MA: Lexington.

Bureau, B. (1993). *Empowerment is more than a buzzword, it's a way of life!* Lawrence, MA: National Empowerment Center.

California Pan-Ethnic Health Network. (1992). *A Multi-Cultural approach to health care system reform.* Berkeley, CA: Author.

California Rural Legal Assistance. (1994). *Farmworkers and national health reform.* San Francisco, CA: Author.

Carrad, J. (1983, October 28). *Morbidity and Mortality Weekly Report,* 554.

Carrillo, C. (1993, April). *Principles for a paradigm shift: Toward a human services policy for Latinos.* Testimony to National Task Force on Health Care Reform, Washington, DC.

Carrillo, J.E. (1991). *The state of the Health and Hospitals Corporation. A report to the HHC board of directors–April 1990 to September 1991.* New York: Health and Hospitals Corporation.

Carrillo, J. E., & De La Cancela, V. (1992). The Cambridge Hospital Latino Health Clinic: A model for interagency integration of health services for Latinos at the provider level. *National Medical Association, 84* (6), 513–519.

Casas, J. (1992). A culturally sensitive model for evaluating alcohol and other drug abuse prevention programs: A Hispanic perspective. In M. A. Orlandi, R. Weston, & L. G. Epstein (Eds.). *Cultural competence for evaluators: A guide for alcohol and other drug abuse prevention practitioners working with ethnic/racial communities* (pp. 75–116). Rockville, MD: Office for Substance Abuse Prevention, U.S. Department of Health and Human Services.

Center for Health Policy Development. (1993, April). *Mexican Americans and other Latinos in the United States: Unique families in need of a quality health care delivery system.* Testimony to National Task Force on Health Care Reform, Washington, DC.

Center on Budget and Policy Priorities. (1988). *Shortchanged: Recent developments in Hispanic poverty, income and employment.* Washington, DC: Center on Budget and Policy Priorities.

Centers for Disease Control. (1993, July). United States AIDS cases reported through June 1993. *HIV/AIDS Surveillance Second Quarter Editions,* 5 (2).

Chang, F. H., & Tang, S. (1977). A neighborhood health center: One community's solution. *Civil Rights Digest,* 19–23.

Chen, M. S. (1994). Health of Pacific Americans/Pacific Islanders. *Asian American and Pacific Islander Journal of Health, 2* (3).

Chen, M. S. (1995). Health status of Chinese Americans: Challenges and opportunities. *Asian American and Pacific Islander Journal of Health, 3* (1), 8–16.

Chin, J. L. (1991). Health care issues for Asian Americans. *Journal of Multi-Cultural Community Health, 1* (2), 17–22.

Chin, J. L. (1992). The right to serve: Barriers to Asian Pacific Islander health provider development; A perspective from community health centers. *Partners in human service: Shaping health care and civil rights policy.* Paper presented at symposium of the Asian American Health Forum. Office of Minority Health, Office for Civil Rights.

Chin, J.L., De La Cancela, V., & Jenkins, Y.M. (1993). *Diversity in psychotherapy: The politics of race, ethnicity, and gender.* Westport, CT: Praeger.

Chrisman, N. (1981). Folk beliefs, popular culture and health. *University of Washington Medicine, 8* (1), 21–28.

Chu, B. (1993, November 15). Testimony before the New York City Council Committee on Health on HHC and the Mayor's Management Report. New York: HHC Office of Intergovernmental Relations.

Clymer, A. (1993, November 14). Growing concerns on covering all, but how? *New York Times.*

Coalition of Hispanic Health and Human Services Organizations. (1991). *Healthy people 2000 objectives and component objectives focusing on*

Hispanic communities: A chartbook. Washington, DC: National Coalition of Hispanic Health and Human Services Organizations.

Coddington, D., Keen, D., et al. (1990). *The alternatives. The crisis in health care.* Jossey-Bass.

Coleman, S. (1996, February 18). An AIDS campaign for black men. *The Boston Sunday Globe,* C-1.

The Commonwealth Fund. (1995). *National comparative survey of minority health care.* New York: Author.

Cook, D., & Webb, L. (1993, April 28). *Health care financing in a changing environment.* Presented at National Association of Health Services Executives Eighth Annual Educational Conference, New Orleans.

Cooper, H. (1993, November 2). If poor can choose, will they pick urban hospitals? *The Wall Street Journal.*

Cornelius, L.J. (1991). Access to medical care for Black Americans with an episode of illness. *Journal of the National Medical Association, 83* (7), 617–626.

Council on Scientific Affairs. (1991). Hispanic health in the United States. *Journal of the American Medical Association, 265* (2), 248–252.

Covey, S. R. (1990). *The seven habits of highly effective people.* New York: Fireside.

Cross, T. L., Bazron, B. J., Dennis, K. W., & Issacs, M. R. (1989). *Towards a culturally competent system of care, Volume I.* Washington, DC: Georgetown University, Children and Adolescent Service Systems Program Technical Assistance Center.

Cummings, C., & DeHart, D. (1995). Ethnic minority physical health: Issues and interventions. In J. F. Aponte, R. Rivers, J. Wohl (Eds.). *Psychological interventions and cultural diversity* (pp. 240–249). Needham Heights, MA: Alyn and Bacon.

Dannemiller, K.D., & Jacobs, R.W. (1992). Changing the way organizations change: A revolution of common sense. *Applied Behavioral Sciences, 28* (4), 480–498.

Davis, A., & Jordan, J. (1994). Foreword. In L. Villarosa (Ed.). *Body and soul* (xi–xii). New York: HarperCollins.

De La Cancela, V. (1978). Culture-specific psychotherapy: Espiritismo, santerismo, curanderismo—an overview. *Proceedings of Fourth Annual Spring Conference of the New York Association of Black Psychologists,* 128–152.

De La Cancela, V. (1986). A critical analysis of Puerto Rican machismo: Implications for clinical practice. *Psychotherapy, 23* (2), 291–296.

De La Cancela, V. (1989a). Minority AIDS prevention: Moving beyond cultural perspectives towards sociopolitical empowerment. *AIDS Education and Prevention, 1* (2), 141–153.

De La Cancela, V. (1989b). Salud, dinero y amor: Beyond wishing Latinos good health. *Practice: Journal of Politics, Economics, Psychology, Sociology, and Culture, 6* (3) & 7 (1), 81–94.

De La Cancela, V. (1990a). Factores psicosociales-culturales en el cuidado de la salud I: Consideraciones generales (Psychosocial-cultural factors in health care I: General considerations). *Medico Interamericano*, August, 23–28.

De La Cancela, V. (1990b). Factores psicosociales-culturales en el cuidado de la salud II: Trastornos comunes (Psychosocial-cultural factors in health care II: Common disorders). *Medico Interamerico*, September, 33–36.

De La Cancela, V. (1991a). The endangered Black male: Reversing the trend for African-American and Latino males. *Journal of Multi-Cultural Community Health*, *1* (1), 10–19.

De La Cancela, V. (1991b). Salsa and control: an ameRican response to Latino health care needs. *Journal of Multi-Cultural Community Health*, *1* (2), 23–29.

De La Cancela, V. (1995a). Companerismo: Urban health and client empowerment through networking. *Focus: Notes from the Society for the Psychological Study of Ethnic Minority Issues, 9* (1), 10–12.

De La Cancela, V. (1995b). Latino/a ATOD prevention research, evaluation and instrumentation: an empowerment perspective. *Proceedings of Second Symposium for Mental Health Professionals of Color*, 51–62.

De La Cancela, V. (1995, September). Mental health and substance abuse prevention in public managed care systems: framing the discussion. Remarks made at the Center for Substance Abuse Prevention sponsored roundtable, entitled *Prevention: An integral part of managed care*, Washington, DC.

De La Cancela, V., Guarnaccia, P.J., & Carrillo, E. (1986). Psychosocial distress among Latinos: A critical analysis of ataques de nervios. *Humanity and Society, 10* (4), 431–446.

De La Cancela, V., Jenkins, Y.M., & Chin, J.L. (1993). Diversity in psychotherapy: Examination of racial, ethnic, gender and political issues. In J.L. Chin, V. De La Cancela & Y.M. Jenkins. *Diversity in psychotherapy: The politics of race, ethnicity, and gender.* Westport, CT: Praeger.

De La Cancela, V., & McDowell, A. (1992). AIDS: Health care intervention models for communities of color. *Journal of Multicultural Social Work, 2* (3), 107–122.

De La Cancela, V., & Sotomayor, G.M. (1993). Rainbow warriors: Reducing institutional racism in mental health. *Journal of Mental Health Counseling, 15* (1), 55–71.

Delgado, J., & Estrada, L. (1992, September 28–30). *Improving data collection strategies.* Paper commissioned for Surgeon General's National Workshop on Hispanic/Latino Health, Washington, DC.

Department of General Services. (1993). *The 1993–94 green book: The official directory of the City of New York.* New York: City Publishing Center.

Dever, G.E. (1989). Migrant health status: Profile of a population with complex health problems. *Migrant Clinicians Network.* Austin, TX: National Migrant Resource Program.

DiMatteo, M. R., & Taranta, A. (1979). Nonverbal community and physician-patient rapport: An empirical study. *Professional Psychology, 10* (4), 540–547.

Duff, K., Garcia-Coll, C., Potter, M., & Stewart, E. (1995). *Meeting the needs of women in prison: Diversity and relationships*. Wellesley, MA: The Stone Center for Developmental Studies and Services.

Ehrenreich, B. (1990, December 10). Our health-care disgrace. *TIME*, 112.

Eisenberg, L. (1992). Treating depression and anxiety in the primary care setting. *Health Affairs, 11* (3), 149–156.

Elders, J. M., Perry, C. L., Eriksen, M. P., & Giovino, G. A. (1994). The report of the surgeon general: Preventing tobacco use among young people. *American Journal of Public Health, 84* (4), 543–547.

Elmhurst Hospital Center. (1993). Managed care comes to Elmhurst Hospital. *Update: A Newsletter for Employees and Friends of Elmhurst Hospital, 7* (4).

Engel, G.L. (1959). "Psychogenic" pain and the pain-prone patient. *American Journal of Medicine, 26*, 899–918.

Fabrega, H., & Tyma, S. (1976). Language and cultural influences in the description of pain. *British Journal of Medical Psychology, 49*, 349–371.

Farb, P., & Armelagos, G. (1980). *Consuming passions: The anthropology of eating*. Boston: Houghton-Mifflin.

Feingold, E. (1994). Health care reform—More than cost containment and universal access. *American Journal of Public Health, 84* (5), 727–728.

Ferguson, R. (1993, January–February). Provider networks and integration: Restructuring health care in Cook County, Illinois. *Outreach, 14* (1).

Flega et al. (1985). Prevalence of diabetes and impaired glucose tolerance in Mexican-Americans, Cubans, and Puerto Ricans, ages 20–74, in the Hispanic health and nutrition examination survey, 1982–1984. Diabetes Working Group, National Center for Health Statistics.

Fordyce, W.E. (1976). *Behavioral methods for chronic pain and illness*. St. Louis, MO: Mosby.

Forman, M., Lu, M.C., Leung, M., & Ponce, N. (1990). *Dispelling the myth of a healthy minority*. San Francisco: Asian American Health Forum.

Frank, R. G., Sullivan, M. J., & DeLeon, P. H. (1994). Health care reform in the states. *American Psychologist, 49* (10), 855–867.

Frank, R. G., & Vandenbos, G. R. (1994). Health care reform: The 1993–1994 evolution. *American Psychologist, 49* (10), 851–853.

Fraser, I., & Tappert, T.N. (1993 January–February). Health care reform: AHA's strategy. *Outreach, 14* (1).

Free Clinic Foundation. (1990). *Directory of free and community clinics in the United States* (1st ed.). Roanoke, VA: Free Clinic Foundation.

Freire, P. (1968). *The pedagogy of the oppressed*. New York: Seabury Press.

Gary, L.E. (1978). Mental health: the problem and the product. In L.E. Gary (Ed.). *Mental health: A challenge to the Black community* (pp. 26–47). Philadelphia: Dorrance.

Gibbs, J.M. (1993, Fall). New York City Health and Hospitals Corporation managed care network development. *The Safety Net*, 4–5.

Ginzberg, E. (1991, January 9). Access to health care for Hispanics. *Journal of the American Medical Association, 265* (2), 238–241.

Glied, S., & Kofman, S. (1995), *Women and mental health: Issues for health reform.* New York: Commonwealth Fund for Women's Health.

Grace, C.A. (1992). Practical considerations for program professionals and evaluators working with African-American communities. In M.A. Orlandi, R. Weston & L.G. Epstein (Eds.). *Cultural competence for evaluators: A guide for alcohol and other drug abuse prevention practitioners working with ethnic/racial communities* (pp. 55–74). Rockville, MD: Office for Substance Abuse Prevention, U.S. Department of Health and Human Services.

Green, L.W., & Kreuter, M.W. (1991). *Health promotion planning: An educational and environmental approach.* Mountain View, CA: Mayfield.

Guarnaccia, P. (1981). Puerto Ricans, asthma, and the healthcare system. *Medical Anthropology Newsletter, 12* (2), 9–17.

Gunatilake, S., & Forouzesh, M.R. (1989–90). Integrating organizational development skills with community organization practice: The key to successful national health care programs. *International Quarterly of Community Health Education, 10* (1), 39–51.

Harden, C.M. (1993, April 29). *Access and indigent care issues: The heart of the health care challenge.* Presented at National Association of Health Services Executives Eighth Annual Educational Conference, New Orleans.

Harrell, S.P. (1995, August 13). Multicultural curriculum content: Integration of multicultural issues into a research course. Presentation at the Annual Convention of the American Psychological Association.

Hawkins, D., & Rosenbaum, S. (1992). *Lives in the balance: A national, state, and county profile of America's medically underserved.* Washington, DC: National Association of Community Health Centers.

Heckler, M. M. (1985). *Report of the Secretary's Task Force on Black and Minority Health.* Washington, DC: U.S. Department of Health and Human Services.

Helman, C.G. (1978). "Feed a cold, starve a fever"—Folk models of infection in an English suburban community, and their relation to medical treatment. *Culture, Medicine and Psychiatry, 1,* 107–137.

Helman, C.G. (1981). Disease versus illness in general practice. *Journal of the Royal College of General Practitioners, 131,* 548–522.

Helman, C.G. (1985). *Health, culture and illness.* Boston: Wright.

Herman, J. (1991). *Trauma and recovery.* New York: Basic Books.

Herrell, I. (1994). *Health care issues affecting the Hispanic population at a time of health care reform.* Committee on Small Business, House of Representatives, Washington, DC: U.S. Government Printing Office.

Herrick, R.R. (1993). Medicaid and managed care. In P.R. Kongstvedt (Ed.). *The managed health care handbook.* Gaithersburg, MD: Aspen.

Hilliard, R.D. (1980). Discussing emotional etiology for illness with medical patients. In M. Jospe, J. Neiberding, & B.D. Cohen (Eds.). *Psychological factors in health care* (pp. 79–83). Lexington, MA: Lexington.

hooks, b. (1994). Living to love. In E. White (Ed.). *The Black woman's health book* (pp. 332–341). Seattle, WA: Seal Press.

Horgan, C. M. (1985). Specialty and general ambulatory mental health services. *Archives of General Psychiatry. 42*, 565–572.

Institute for Puerto Rican Policy. (1994, June). Puerto Ricans and other Latinos in the United States: March 1993. *IPR Datanote*, 16.

Iscoe, I. (1974). Community psychology and the competent community. *American Psychologist, 29* (8), 607–613.

Issacs, M., & Benjamin, M. (1991). South Cove Community Health Center. *Towards a culturally competent system of care, Volume II.* Washington, DC: Georgetown University, Children and Adolescent Service Systems Program Technical Assistance Center.

Jemmott, L., & Jemmott, J. (1991). Applying the theory of reasoned action to AIDS risk behavior: Condom use among Black men. *Nursing Research, 48*, 228–234.

Jenkins, Y. (1995). Diversity and perceptions. In K. Duff, C. Garcia-Coll, M. Potter, & E. Stewart. *Meeting the needs of women in prison: Diversity and relationships.* Wellesley, MA. The Stone Center for Developmental Studies and Services.

Jenkins, Y. M., De La Cancela, V., & Chin, J. L. (1993). Three historical overviews. In J. L. Chin, V. De La Cancela & Y. M. Jenkins *Diversity in psychotherapy* (pp. 17–44). Westport, CT: Praeger.

Jennings, J. (1994). Poverty and power. *Boston Review, 19* (3&4).

Jereb, J.A., Kelly, G.D., Dooley, S.W., et al. (1991). Tuberculosis morbidity in the United States: Final data, 1990. *Morbidity and Mortality Weekly Report, 40*, (No.55–3), 23–26.

Jordan, J. (1984). Empathy and self boundaries. *Work in progress*, 16. Wellesley, MA: Wellesley College, Stone Center Working Paper Series.

Jordan, J.B., Kaplan, A., Miller, J. B., Stiver, I., & Surrey, J.L. (1991). *Women's growth in connection.* New York: Guilford.

Jospe, M., Nieberding, J., & Cohen, B.D. (Eds.). (1980). *Psychological factors in health care.* Lexington, MA: Lexington.

Kaplan, E., & Brandeau, M. (1994). AIDS policy modeling by example. *AIDS, 8* (1), S333–S340.

Katon, W., Kleinman, A., & Rosen, G. (1982). Depression and somatization: A review. Part I. *American Journal of Medicine, 72*, 127–135.

Katon, W., Kleinman, A., & Rosen, G. (1982). Depression and somatization: A review. Part II. *American Journal of Medicine, 72*, 241–247.

Kemnitzer, L. (1980). Cultural background of Native American health behavior. In M. Jospe, J. Nieberding, & B.D. Cohen (Eds.). *Psychological factors in health care* (pp. 347–363). Lexington, MA: Lexington.

Kiev, A. (1972). *Transcultural psychiatry.* New York: Free Press.

Kim, S., McLeod, J.H., & Shantzis, C. (1992). Cultural competence for evaluators working with Asian-American communities: Some practical considerations. In M.A. Orlandi, R. Weston, & L.G. Epstein (Eds.). *Cultural competence for evaluators: A guide for alcohol and other drug abuse prevention practitioners working with ethnic/racial communities* (pp. 203–260). Rockville, MD: Office for Substance Abuse Prevention, U.S. Department of Health and Human Services.

Kleinman, A. (1980). *Patients and healers in the context of culture.* Berkeley: University of California Press.

Kleinman, A. (1988). *Rethinking psychiatry: From cultural category to personal experiences.* New York: Free Press

Kleinman, A. (1996). *Writing at the margin: Discourse between anthropology and medicine.* Berkeley: University of California Press.

Kleinman, A., Eisenberg, L., & Good, B. (1978). Clinical lessons from anthropologic and cross cultural research. *Annals of Internal Medicine, 88,* 251–258.

Knapp, P.H. (1977). Psychotherapeutic management of bronchial asthma. In E. Wittkower & H. Warnes (Eds.) *Psychosomatic medicine: Its clinical applications* (pp. 347–363). Hagerstown, MD: Harper & Row.

Koh, H.K., & Koh, H.C. (1993). Health issues in Korean Americans. *Asian American and Pacific Islander Journal of Health, 1* (2), 176–194.

Kolata, G. (1991, March 10). In medical research equal opportunity doesn't always apply. *New York Times.*

Kongstvedt, P.R. (1993a). Changing provider behavior in managed care plans. In P.R. Kongstvedt (Ed.). *The managed health care handbook.* Gaithersburg, MD: Aspen.

Kongstvedt, P.R. (1993b). Primary care in open panels. In P.R. Kongstvedt (Ed.). *The managed health care handbook.* Gaithersburg, MD: Aspen.

Kwiatkowski, C., & Maislen, S. (1991). New York State's mandatory managed care model. *Journal of Multi-Cultural Community Health, 1* (2), 34–39.

Labonte, R. (1994). *Health promotion and empowerment: Practice frameworks.* Toronto, Canada: Center for Health Promotion.

Landy, D., (Ed.). (1977). *Culture, disease and healing studies in medical anthropology.* New York: Macmillan.

Latino Coalition for a Healthy California. (1992). *A Latino perspective on access to care and health system reform.* San Francisco: Author.

Latino Coalition for a Healthy California. (1993). *The American health security act: A Latino perspective. A preliminary analysis.* San Francisco: Author.

Latino Coalition for a Healthy California. (1994a). *The health security act: A Latino perspective.* San Francisco: Author.

Latino Coalition for a Healthy California. (1994b). *Proposed amendments to health care reform bills.* San Francisco: Author.

Latino Health News. (1994, January). Health conditions of California's Latino population. *Latino Health News.*

Lazare, A. (1973). Hidden conceptual models in clinical psychiatry. *New England Journal of Medicine, 288* (7), 345–351.

Lefebvre, R., & Flora, J. (1988). Social marketing and public health intervention. *Health Education Quarterly, 15,* 299–315.

Leviton, L. (1995). Integrating psychology and public health. *American Psychologist, 51* (1), 42–51.

Leviton, L., Chen, H., Marsh, G., & Talbott, E. (1993). Evaluation issues in the Drake Chemical Workers Notification and Health Registry Study. *American Journal of Industrial Medicine, 23,* 197–204.

Lin-Fu, J.S. (1993). Asian and Pacific Islander Americans: An overview of demographic characteristics and health care issues. *Asian American and Pacific Islander Journal of Health, 1* (1), 20–35.

Littlewood, R., & Lipsedge, M. (1982). *Aliens and alienists.* Harmondsworth: Penguin.

Lohman, P. (1993). Information is everything. *Prospectus, 2,* 4.

Low, S. (1981). The meaning of nervios. *Culture, Medicine and Psychiatry, 5,* 350–357.

Ludwig, A.M. (1982). "Nerves:" a sociomedical diagnosis...of sorts. *American Journal of Psychotherapy, 36* (3), 350–357.

Luna, G.C., & Rotheram-Borus, M.J. (1995). The limitations of empowerment programs for young people living with HIV. *American Journal of Community Psychology, 5.*

MacLeod, G.K. (1994). An overview of managed health care. In P.R. Kongstvedt (Ed.). *The managed health care handbook.* Gaithersburg, MD: Aspen.

Majors, R., & Billson, J. (1992). *Cool pose.* New York: Lexington Books.

Marin, G., Amaro, H., Eisenberg, C., & Opava-Stitzer, S. (1992, September 28–30). *The development of a relevant and comprehensive research agenda to improve Hispanic health.* Paper commissioned for Surgeon General's National Workshop on Hispanic/Latino Health, Washington, DC.

Marmot, M. (1981). Culture and illness: Epidemiological evidence. In M.J. Christie & P.G. Mellet (Eds.). *Foundations of psychosomatics* (pp. 323–340). Chichester: John Wiley.

Matarazzo, J.D. (1984). Behavioral immunogens and pathogens in health and illness. In B.L Hammonds & C.J. Scheirer (Eds.). *Psychology and Health: Master Lecture Series* (pp. 5–44). Washington, DC: American Psychological Association.

Matthews, K.A., Shumaker, S.A., Bowen, D. J., Langer, R.D., Hunt, J.R., Kaplan, R.M., Klesges, R.C., & Ritenbaugh, C. (1997). Women's Health Initiative: Why now? What is it? What's new? *American Psychologist, 52* (2), 101–113.

Matthews, A., & Ridgeway, V. (1984). Psychological preparation for surgery. In A. Steptoe & A. Matthews (Eds.). *Health care and behavior* (pp. 231–259). London: Academic.

Mayeno, L., & Hirota, S. M. (1990). Access to health care. In N.W.S. Zane, D.T. Takeuchi, & K.N.J. Young (Eds.). *Confronting critical health issues of Asian and Pacific Islander Americans* (pp. 3–21). Thousand Oaks, CA: Sage.

Mays, V., & Cohran, S. (1988). Issues in the perception of AIDS risk reduction activities by Black and Hispanic/Latina women. *American Psychologist, 43,* 949–957.

McAlister, A. (1991). Population behavior change: A theory-based approach. *Journal of Public Health Policy, 12,* 345–361.

McKeown, C.T., Rubenstein, R.A., & Kelley, J.G. (1987). Anthropology, the meaning of community, and prevention. In L.A. Jason, R.E. Hess, R.D.

Felner, & J.N. Moritsuga (Eds.). Prevention. Toward a multidisciplinary approach. *Prevention in Human Services, 5* (2). New York: Haworth Press.

McKusick, L. (1991, April). *HIV Frontline*, No. 1.

McKusick, L. (1991, May). *HIV Frontline*, No. 2.

McNamee, M. (1993, August 30). Snickers and sniping at Clinton from the left. *Business Week*, 35.

Mechanic, D. (1990). Treating mental illness: Generalist versus specialist. *Health Affairs*, 61–75.

Medicaid Working Group. (1993). *Developing managed care for people with disabilities and chronic illness: Issues and strategies.* Boston: Medicaid Working Group.

Mezzich J., Kleinman, A., Fabrega, H., & Parrone, D. (Eds.) (1996). *Culture and psychiatric diagnosis.* Washington, DC: American Psychiatric Press.

Miller, J. B. (1976). *Toward a new psychology of women.* Boston: Beacon Press.

Miller, J. B. (1986). What do we mean by relationships? *Work in progress, 22.* Wellesley, MA: Wellesley College, Stone Center Working Paper Series.

Minkler, M., & Cox, K. (1980). Creating critical consciousness in health: Applications of Freire's philosophy and methods to the health care setting. *International Journal of Health Services, 10* (2), 311–322.

Molina, C.W., & Aguirre-Molina, M. (Eds.). (1994). *Latino health in the US: A growing challenge.* Washington, DC: The American Public Health Association.

Munoz, R.F. (1983). *Prevention intervention research: A challenge to minority researchers.* Presentation at the NIMH Technical Assistance Workshop on Prevention Intervention Research: Special Population Groups.

Nathanson, S.N. (1993, January–February). A Chicago consortium: Working with physicians to provide care to the underserved. *Outreach, 14* (1).

National Association of Community Health Centers. (1995). *America's health centers: Accessible, efficient providers of quality health care for underserved people and communities.* Washington, DC: Author.

National Boricua Health Organization. (1990). *National Boricua Health Organization. By laws and national constitution.* Newark, NJ: Forest Hills Family Associates.

National Hispanic Health Policy Summit. (1992, April 8). *Summary of discussions and recommendations in assessing Hispanic health needs.*

Navarro, V. (1994). The future of public health in health care reform. *American Journal of Public Health, 84* (5), 729–730.

New York City Health and Hospitals Corporation. (1989). *Strategic directions for the year 2000: A staff working paper.* New York: HHC Office of Strategic Planning.

New York City Health and Hospitals Corporation. (1992). *Child and adolescent health services: A guide to referral resources.* New York: HHC Office of Primary Care Development.

New York City Health and Hospitals Corporation. (1993a). *An introduction to managed care, Medicaid managed care, and Communicare*. New York: Office of Managed Care Education and Special Projects.

New York City Health and Hospitals Corporation. (1993b). *President Clinton's health security plan: What it means for safety-net providers and underserved communities*. New York: HHC Office of Intergovernmental Relations.

New York City Health and Hospitals Corporation. (1993c). *A strategic direction for the Health and Hospitals Corporation: Update of the HHC strategic plan*. New York: HHC Office of Strategic Planning.

New York City Health and Hospitals Corporation. (1993d). *Strategic planning retreat. Office of Primary Care Services/Alternative Delivery Systems. June 30*. New York: HHC Office of Primary Care Services.

New York City Health and Hospitals Corporation. (1994a). *Helping you spread the word: A facilitator's guide to marketing managed care*. New York: Office of Managed Care Education and Special Projects.

New York City Health and Hospitals Corporation. (1994b). *Managed care made easy: A question and answer guide to managed health care*. New York: Office of Managed Care and Special Projects.

New York City Health and Hospitals Corporation. (1994c). *Managed care "101" learning activities and general overview*. New York: Office of Managed Care Education and Special Projects.

New York City Health and Hospitals Corporation. (1994d). *Reaching the customer: A sales representative's guide to selling the Metropolitan Health Plan*. New York: Office of Managed Care Education and Special Projects.

New York City Health and Hospitals Corporation. (1994e). *The three main issues for providers of the underserved in federal health care reform*. New York: Office of Intergovernmental Relations, April.

New York City Planning Commission. (1993, December). City Planning releases socioeconomic study of Puerto Rican New Yorkers. *City Planning News*.

New York State Department of Social Services. (1993). *New York State Medicaid Managed Care annual report and state plan*. New York: Department of Social Services.

Nicot, J., & Colon, E. (1990). *A call to action IV*. New York: Association of Puerto Rican Executive Directors.

Nieves, S. (1994). Betraying the children: The "New" Board of Education. *Critica: A Journal of Puerto Rican Policy & Politics, 2*, 1, 12–13.

Nobbe, G. (1993). Urban medicine: The hope of the future. *Medical Herald, 2* (10), 1–8.

O'Connor, J. (1975). Social and cultural factors influencing drinking behavior. *Irish Journal of Medical Science, 1*, 65–71.

Orlandi, M.A. (1992). The challenge of evaluating community-based prevention programs: A cross-cultural perspectiveIn M.A. Orlandi, R. Weston, & L.G. Epstein (Eds.). *Cultural competence for evaluators: A guide for alcohol and other drug abuse prevention practitioners working with eth-*

nic/racial communities (pp. 1–22). Rockville, MD: Office for Substance Abuse Prevention, U.S. Department of Health and Human Services.

Ortiz, H. (1993). *Salud means health.* Presented to Hilary Rodham Clinton, Chairperson, White House Task Force on Health Reform by National Congress for Puerto Rican Rights, April 14, Washington, DC.

Overall, N. A., & Williamson, J. (1988). *Community oriented primary care in action: A practice manual for primary care settings.* (Contract No. 240–84-0124). Washington, DC: U.S. Department of Health and Human Services, Public Health Service.

Patton, L. T. (1990). *Community health centers: A working bibliography.* Washington, DC: National Association of Community Health Centers.

Pear, R. (1993, November 14). A.M.A. challenges the President's plan. *New York Times.*

Perez, S.M. (1994). Puerto Ricans and the politics of welfare reform. *Critica: A Journal of Puerto Rican Policy & Politics*, August, *3*, 1, 6–7.

Petrovich, J. (1987). *Northeast Hispanic needs. A guide for action.* Washington, DC: ASPIRA Institute for Policy Research.

Pinderhughes, E. B. (1989). *Understanding race, ethnicity, and power.* New York: The Free Press.

Plaska, M., & Vieth, E. A. (1995). The community health center: An enduring model for the past and future. *The Journal of Ambulatory Care Management, 18* (2), 3–8.

Posner, T. (1980). Ritual in the surgery. *MIMS Magazine*, August 1, 41–48.

Pulse Collective. (1990, Summer). Health & Hospitals Corporation, New York City. 20 years of struggle. *Pulse: A Newsletter for Workers and Activists in Health, 5* (1).

Racer, H.J. (1980). Psychological medicine and family practice. In M. Jospe, J. Nieberding, & B.D. Cohen (Eds.). *Psychological factors in health care* (pp. 323–340). Lexington, MA: Lexington.

Relman, A.S. (1992, March). What market values are doing to medicine. *The Atlantic Monthly*, 99–106.

Relman, A.S. (1993, October 23). Doctors can learn to help control health costs. *New York Newsday.*

Relman, A.S. (1993, November 17). Patients can't play with the health market. *New York Newsday.*

Rendon, M. (1984). Myths and stereotypes in minority groups. *International Journal of Social Psychology, 30* (4), 297–309.

Richie, B. E. (1992, Fall). *Community organizing for health.* Course presented at Program in Community Health Education, Hunter College School of Health Sciences, New York, NY.

Rogers, E.M. (1983). *Diffusion of innovations.* New York: Free Press.

Rosado, J.W. (1980). Important psychocultural factors in the delivery of mental health services to lower-class Puerto Rican clients: A review of recent studies. *Journal of Community Psychology, 8*, 215–226.

Rosen, G., Kleinman, A., & Katon, W. (1982). Somatization in family practice: A biopsychosocial approach. *The Journal of Family Practice, 14* (3), 493–502.

Rosenbaum, S. (1987). *Community and migrant health centers: Two decades of achievement.* Washington, DC: National Association of Community Health Centers.

Rosenthal, E. (1993, November 14). Lack of doctors for the poor is obstacle to health plans. *New York Times.*

Russell, L. (1985). *Is prevention better than cure?* Washington, DC: Brookings Institution.

Rowley, D.L., Hogue, C.J.R., Blackmore, C.A., Ferre, C.D., Hatfield-Timajchy, K., Branch, P., & Atrash, H.K. (1993). Preterm delivery among African-American Women: A research strategy. *American Journal of Preventive Medicine, 9* (6), 1–6.

Ryan, W. (1976). *Blaming the victim.* New York: Vintage Books.

Sagara, C., & Kiang, P. (1992). *Recognizing poverty in Boston's Asian American community.* Boston: The Boston Persistent Poverty Project.

Salas Rojas, A. (1992, January 14). Latinos fight against AIDS. *New York Newsday.*

Scheffler, R., & Radany, M.H. (1990). *The financing of public mental health care in California: Overview and research agenda.* Berkeley, CA: Institute of Mental Health Services Research.

Schur, C.L., Bernstein, A.B., & Berk M. L. (1987). The importance of distinguishing Hispanic subpopulations in the use of medical care. *Medical Care, 25* (7), 627–641.

Scott, C.S. (1974). Health and healing practices among five ethnic groups in Miami, Florida. *Public Health Reports, 89* (6), 524–532.

Scott, G. (1993, October 26). City hospitals told of $ threat. *New York Newsday.*

Sharfstein, S. S., Stoline, A. M., & Goldman, H. H. (1993). Psychiatric care and health insurance reform. *American Journal of Psychiatry, 150* (1).

Sheola, R.A. (1994). *Testimony before the New York City Council Committee on Health, November 4.* New York: HHC Office of Managed Care, Planning and Marketing.

Sifontes, J.F., & Mayol, P.M. (1976). Bronchial asthma in Puerto Rican children. *Boletín de la Asociación Médica de Puerto Rico, 68,* 336–339.

Sisk, J.E., Gorman, S., & Carr, W. (1993, May). *Medicaid managed care in New York City: A survey of the enrolled and non-enrolled population.* Proposal to Commonwealth Fund by Columbia University School of Public Health, New York.

Smith, D.R., & Anderson, R.J. (1990). Community-responsive medicine: A call for a new academic discipline. *Journal of Health Care for the Poor and Underserved, 1* (2), 219–227

Smith, D.R., Brooks, D.D., & Anderson, R.J. (1991). The involution of medicine—A study of catastrophic health polices for preventive strategies. *Lyceum Journal, 8* (1), 7–11.

Smith, G. R., & Burns, B. J. (1993). Recommendations of the Little Rock working group on mental and chemical dependency disorders in health-care reform. *Journal of Mental Health Administration, 20* (3), 247–252.

Smith, K. Living in the age of AIDS. (1995, December) *Essence*, 64.

Smith, M. (1991). Problems confronting Blacks. *HIV Frontline*, 2, 5.

Snook, I.D. (1992). *Hospitals: What they are and how they work.* Gaithersburg, MD: Aspen.

Snow, L.F. (1978). Sorcerers, saints and charlatans: Black folk healers in urban America. *Culture, Medicine and Psychiatry*, 2, 69–106.

Sotomayor, G.M. (1985, August). *Latina teenagers and chemical dependency.* Paper presented at Illinois Alcoholism and Drug Dependence Association and Illinois Women and Substance Abuse Coalition Annual Conference, Springfield, IL.

Source Collective. (1974). *Organizing for health care: A tool for change.* Boston, MA: Beacon.

South Cove Community Health Center. (1994, June). *Health care reform: Impact for Asian Americans.* Community Forum cosponsored by South Cove Community Health Center and U.S. Public Health Service, Region I, Office of Minority Health.

Starfield, B. (1992). *Primary care.* New York: Oxford University Press.

Sue, D. W. (1992). Multiculturalism: The road less traveled. *American Counselor*, 1, 6–14.

Suinn, R.M. (1996). The case for psychological services in primary health care: Medical costs offset. *Public Service Psychology*, 21 (1), 14.

Surrey, J. (1991a). Relationship and empowerment. In J.B. Jordan, A. Kaplan, J. B. Miller, I. Stiver, & J.L. Surrey. *Women's growth in connection* (pp. 162–180). New York: Guilford.

Surrey, J.L. (1991b). The self-in-relation: A theory of women's development. In J.B. Jordan, A. Kaplan, J.B. Miller, I. Stiver & J.L. Surrey. *Women's growth in connection* (pp. 51–66). New York: Guilford.

Surrey, J. (1995). Women in prisons and substance abuse: A relational perspective. In K. Duff, C. Garcia-Coll, M. Potter, & E. Stewart (Eds.). *Meeting the needs of women in prison: Diversity and relationships* (p. 20). Wellesley, MA: The Stone Center for Developmental Studies and Services.

Susser, M. (1994). The logic in ecological: I. The logic of analysis. *American Journal of Public Health*, 84 (5), 825–829.

Szapocznik, J. (1994). Epilogue. In J.Szapocznik (Ed.). *A Hispanic/Latino family approach to substance abuse prevention* (pp. 205–207). Rockville, MD: Center for Substance Abuse Prevention, U.S. Department of Health and Human Services.

Szasz, T. (1957). *Pain and pleasure.* New York: Basic Books.

Tafoya, T. (1991). Testing for HIV in Native American communities: Special considerations. *HIV Frontline*, 2, 7.

Takeuchi, D.T., & Young, K.N.J. (1990). Overview of Asian and Pacific Islander Americans. In N.W.S. Zane, D.T. Takeuchi, & K.N.J. Young (Eds.). *Confronting critical health issues of Asian and Pacific Islander Americans* (pp. 3–21). Thousand Oaks, CA: Sage.

Tefft, B. M., & Simeonsson, R. J. (1979). Psychology and the creation of health care settings. *Professional Psychology*, 10 (4), 558–570.

Torrey, E.F. (1968). Psychiatric services for Mexican Americans. Unpublished manuscript.

Trader, H.P. (1977). Survival strategies for oppressed minorities. *Social Work, 22* (1), 10–13.

Tyler, F.B., Brome, D.R., & Williams, J.E. (1991). *Ethnic validity, ecology, and psychotherapy.* New York: Plenum.

UCLA Center for Health Policy Research. (1995). *Women's health-related behaviors and use of clinical preventive services.* New York: The Commonwealth Fund.

United Hospital Fund. (1993). *The state of New York City's municipal hospital system: Report of the City Hospital Visiting Committee.* New York: Author.

United Hospital Fund. (1994). *The state of New York City's municipal hospital system. Report of the City Hospital Visiting Committee.* New York: Author.

U.S. Bureau of the Census. (1993). *Statistical abstract of the United States.* (113th ed.). Washington, DC: U.S. Government Printing Office.

U.S. Department of Health and Human Services. (1985). *Report of the Secretary's Task Force on Black and Minority Health, I.* Executive Summary.

U.S. Department of Health and Human Services. (1991). *Strategies to control tobacco use in the United States: A blueprint for public health action in the 1990s.* Publication No. 92-3316. Washington, DC: National Institutes of Health.

Valdez, R.B., Giachello, A., Rodriguez-Trias, H., Gomez, P., & de la Rocha, C. (1992, September). *Improving access to health care in Hispanic/Latino communities.* Presented at Surgeon General's National Workshop on Hispanic Latino Health: Implementation strategies, Washington, DC.

Velez, P., & Moshipur, J. (1993). To the staff of Elmhurst Hospital. *Update: A Newsletter for Employees and Friends of Elmhurst Hospital, 7* (4), 1.

Ventura, S.J. (1987). Births of Hispanic parentage, 1983 and 1984. *National Center for Health Statistics Monthly Vital Statistics Report, 36* (4) Supplement, (PHS) 87-1120.

Villarosa, L. (Ed.). (1994). *Body and soul.* New York: HarperCollins.

Walker, P.F. (1994, July/August). Delivering culturally competent care in a multicultural society: Challenges for physicians. *HCMS Bulletin,* 8–10.

Wallis, L. A. (1992). Why a curriculum in women's health? *Journal of Women's Health, 21* (1), 55–59.

Washington, H. (1995, January). Examining health care reform. The stakes are high for Black doctors and hospitals. *Emerge,* (IV), 38–39.

Waxler, N.L. (1977). Is mental illness cured in traditional societies? A theoretical analysis. *Culture, Medicine and Psychiatry, 1,* 233–253.

Webb, W.L. (1983). Chronic pain. *Psychosomatics, 1,* 1053–1063.

Weinstein, S., & Stason, W. (1976). *Hypertension: A policy perspective.* Cambridge, MA: Harvard University Press.

Wells, J., Howard, G., Nowlin, W., & Vargas, M. (1986). Presurgical anxiety and postsurgical pain and adjustment: Effects of a stress inoculation procedure. *Journal of Consulting and Clinical Psychology, 54,* 831–835.

Wertlieb, D. (1979). A preventive health paradigm for health care psychologists. Professional Psychology, 10 (4), 548–557.

Whalen, V., Tormala, W., & Osborne, J. (1976, October 20). Critical consciousness for public health care consumers. Paper presented at the 109th annual meeting of the American Public Health Association.

Whigham-Desir, M. (1994, July). Will black doctors win or lose in health reform? Black Enterprise, 70–78.

Wilkenfeld, L. (1994). Staff adjustment to organizational change in a hospital setting: A case example. Psychotherapy Bulletin, 29 (3), 40–44.

Wolf Dresp, C.S. (1985, March). Nervios as culture-bound syndrome among Puerto Rican women. Smith College Studies in Social Work, 115–136.

Wolff, T. (n.d.). Coalition building: One path to empowered communities, Amherst, MA: AHEC/Community Partners.

Yu, E.S.H., & Liu, W.T. (1994). Methodological issues. In N.W.S. Zane, D.T. Takeuchi, & K.N.J. Young (Eds.). Confronting critical health issues of Asian and Pacific Islander Americans (pp. 22–52). Thousand Oaks, CA: Sage.

Zane, N.S.W., Takeuchi, D.T., & Young, K.N.J. (Eds.). (1994). Confronting critical health issues of Asian and Pacific Islander Americans. Thousand Oaks, CA: Sage.

Zola, I.K. (1966). Culture and symptoms. An analysis of patient's presenting complaints. American Sociological Review, 31, 615–630.

Notes on Contributors

Victor De La Cancela, Ph.D., M.P.H., FPPR is a Puerto Rican clinical-community psychologist at Comprehensive Habilitation Services (NY), Clinical Administrator at Gateway Counseling Center (NY), Assistant Clinical Professor of Medical Psychology at College of Physicians and Surgeons, Columbia University and President of Salud Management Associates, an association of independent behavioral healthcare/management consultants and practices. Dr. De La Cancela has previously served as Senior Vice President for Community Health and Primary Care Development, New York City Health and Hospitals Corporation, President of the National Hispanic Psychological Association, and Commissioner, APA Commission of Ethnic Minority Recruitment, Retention and Training in Psychology. He is a Fellow of the American Psychological Association and a Board Certified, Diplomate-Fellow Prescribing Psychologist. His recent publications include *Diversity in psychotherapy: The politics of race, ethnicity, and genter.* Dr. De La Cancela's professional interests include AIDS, substance abuse and alchoholism prevention and training, community-based health and human services management, multicultural workforce development and diversity consultation, community health education and empowerment.

J. Emilio Carrillo, M.D., M.P.H. is a national leader in the development of primary care services and Latino(a) physician development. He has conducted community-based research on smoking and low birth weight prevention as well as cross cultural health care. As

President of New York City's Health and Hospitals Corporation, he reengineered the nation's largest municipal health care network into a primary care centered system. He is the Medical Director of The New York Hospital Community Health Plan.

Jean Lau Chin, Ed.D. is an Asian female psychologist with over 20 years of clinical-administrative experience in mental health and health care. Dr. Chin's administrative background includes co-Director of a child guidance clinic for over 8 years and Executive Director, South Cove Community Health Center (Boston, MA) for the past 6 years. Her recent publications include *Diversity in psychotherapy: The politics of race, ethnicity, and gender* and *Transference and empathy in Asian American psychotheraopy: Cultural values and treatment needs*. Dr. Chin's professional interests include diversity and cultural competence in delivery of community-based health/mental health services, psychotherapy training and administration.

G. Rita Dudley Grant, Ph.D., M.P.H. is formerly Director of the Center for Multicultural Training in Psychology in Boston, MA, and subsequently Assistant Commissioner of Health in the U.S. Virgin Islands. She is currently Clinical Psychologist and Program Developer for V.I. Behavioral Services in the Virgin Islands.

Tessie Guillermo is the Executive Director of the Asian and Pacific Islander American Health Forum, a national health advocacy and policy organization based in San Francisco, California. She currently serves as co-chair of the California Pan Ethnic Health Network, and served two terms on the California Department of Health Services (CDHS) Task Force on Multicultural Health. Through her involvement in both groups, she was instrumental in developing the CDHS's Cultural and Linguistics Standards for its MediCal (California's Medicaid plan) Managed Care Expansion.

Bertha Garrett Holliday, Ph.D. is a community psychologist with interests in family and child socialization, mental health, and social policy. Her professional evolution includes positions as an administrator in the Model Cities program, a university teacher and researcher, a congressional fellow, a national manager of program evaluation in a nonprofit youth-serving organization, and a chief of program evaluation at a state mental health agency. Currently, Dr. Holliday is the Director of Ethnic Minority Affairs at the American Psychological Association in Washington, DC.

Yvonne M. Jenkins, Ph.D. is an African American psychologist at Harvard University Health Services, faculty member of the Jean Baker Miller Training Institute of the Stone Center at Wellesley College, network member of the Center for Multicultural Training in Psychology (Boston, MA) and in private practice with Frauenhofer Psychological Associates (Brookline, MA). Her recent publications include *Diversity in psychotherapy: The politics of race, ethnicity, and gender.* Dr. Jenkins' professional interests include social diversity issues and mental health, college mental health, and women's mental health.

Herbert M. Joseph, Jr., Ph.D., M.P.H. is the Chief Psychologist and Director of the Center for Multicultural Training in Psychology (CMTP) in the Division of Psychiatry at the Boston Medical Center. CMTP's predecessor, the Minority Training Program (MTP) in Clinical and Community Psychology at Boston City Hospital was one of the first sites in the country devoted to training pre-and postdoctoral psychology trainees from racial/ethnic and culturally diverse backgrounds to work in urban, community-based settings in the public sector. An assistant professor of psychiatry at the Boston University School of Medicine, Dr. Joseph's professional interests include child mental health, multicultural training, and public health policy, interventions, and program development in communities of color.

Nancy J. Kennedy, Dr.P.H. has over 25 years of professional and personal experience in the fields of mental health and substance abuse. She is currently the Director of the Office of Managed Care for the Federal Center for Substance Abuse Prevention, a center within the Substance Abuse and Mental Health Services Administration. Dr. Kennedy has functioned in many capacities, having trained health educators at a university and also worked as an epidemiologist at the National Institute on Drug Abuse.

Arthur Kleinman, M.D. is Presley Professor of Medical Anthropology and Psychiatry, Departments of Anthropology and Social Medicine, Harvard University and Chairman, Department of Social Medicine, Harvard Medical School and The Cambridge Hospital.

Ford H. Kuramoto, D.S.W. is National Director of the National Asian Pacific American Families Against Substance Abuse, Inc. (NAPAFASA) in Los Angeles. Dr. Kuramoto has been a direct service worker, supervisor, and manager in both the public and private sectors. He is a licensed clinical social worker and on the editorial board of the American Orthopsychiatric Association Journal.

Jane S. Lin-Fu, M.D., FAAP is Chief, Genetic Service Branch, Maternal and Child Health Bureau, Health Resource Administration, U.S.

Department of Health and Human Services. Dr. Lin-Fu is also the nation's leading expert on childhood lead poisoning and has received the Superior Service Award, the U.S. Public Health Service's highest honor for a civilian. She is widely recognized as a pioneer in the Asian Pacific Islander American health movement.

Carlos Molina, Ed.D. is Professor of Public Health Education at York College, The City University of New York. Dr. Molina also served as the Executive Director of Lincoln Hospital from 1990 to 1992. He is currently an Executive Board Member of the American Public Health Association.

Deborah Prothrow-Stith, M.D., a former Commissioner of the Massachusetts Department of Public Health, is currently Professor of Public Health Practice and Associate Dean for Faculty Development at the Harvard School of Public Health. Dr. Prothrow-Stith is widely known for her violence prevention public health programming and advocacy at the community and local government level.

Pamela Jumper Thurman, Ph.D. is a Research Associate with the Tri-Ethnic Center for Prevention Research, Colorado State University, in Fort Collins, Colorado. Dr. Thurman has conducted research on mental health, violence, community readiness, and substance abuse in Native American communities and provided treatment, evaluation, and consulting services for underserved rural and reservation populations.

Henry Tomes, Ph.D. is the Executive Director of the Public Interest Directorate at the American Psychological Association in Washington, D.C. Dr. Tomes served as Commissioner of the Department of Mental Health for the Commonwealth of Massachusetts.

Rueben C. Warren, D.D.S., Dr.P.H. is the Associate Administrator for Urban Affairs at the Agency for Toxic Substances and Disease Registry (ATSDR) in Atlanta, Georgia, where he has lead agency responsibility for Environmental Justice, Brownfields and Minority Health. From 1988 to 1997, Dr. Warren served as Associate Director for Minority Health at the Centers for Disease Control and Prevention. Dr. Warren served as dean and associate professor of the School of Dentistry, Department of Preventive Dentistry and Community Health, at Meharry Medical College in Nashville, Tennessee. Currently, he is a Clinical Professor, Department of Preventive Medicine and Community Health, Morehouse School of Medicine and Adjunct Professor, Department of Behavioral Sciences and Health Education, Rollins School of Public Health, Emory University, both in Atlanta, Georgia.

Index